DATE DUE

DEMCO 38-296

A PSYCHOLOGICAL APPROACH
TO HOSPITAL-ACQUIRED INFECTIONS

A PSYCHOLOGICAL APPROACH
TO HOSPITAL-ACQUIRED INFECTIONS

C. A. Bartzokas
Emma E. Williams
P. D. Slade

Studies in Health and Human Services
Volume 24

The Edwin Mellen Press
Lewiston/Queenston/Lampeter

Library of Congress Cataloging-in-Publication Data

Bartzokas, C. A. (Chris A.)
    A psychological approach to hospital-acquired infections / C.A.
Bartzokas, Emma E. Williams, P.D. Slade.
    p.   cm.
    Includes bibliographical references and index.
    ISBN 0-7734-9030-2
    1. Nosocomial infections--Prevention--Psychological aspects.
I. Williams, Emma E.   II. Slade, Peter D.   III. Title.
RA969.B377   1994
614.4'4--dc20   94-27126
                                                                              CIP

This is volume 24 in the continuing series
Studies in Health and Human Services
Volume 24 ISBN 0-7734-9030-2
SHHS Series ISBN 0-88946-126-0

A CIP catalog record for this book is available from the British Library.

The Edwin Mellen Press   The Edwin Mellen Press
        Box 450   Box 67
Lewiston, New York   Queenston, Ontario
USA 14092-0450   CANADA L0S 1L0

The Edwin Mellen Press, Ltd.
Lampeter, Dyfed, Wales
UNITED KINGDOM SA48 7DY

Printed in the United States of America

DEDICATION

This monograph is dedicated to Ignaz Philipp Semmelweis (1818 - 1865)

The Progenitor of Infection Control

AUTHORS

Chris A. Bartzokas   is the Consultant in Medical Microbiology & Infection Control, (*Wirral Hospital NHS Trust, Clatterbridge Hospital, Bebington, Wirral, L63 4JY, UK*) and Clinical Lecturer at the University of Liverpool.

Emma E. Williams   is the Forensic Clinical Psychologist, department of Clinical Psychology (*Fairmile Hospital, Wallingford, Oxfordshire OV10 9HH, UK*). Part of the work presented in this monograph has been submitted as a Ph.D. at the University of Liverpool in 1987.

Peter D. Slade   is the Professor of Clinical Psychology, Department of Clinical Psychology, (*University of Liverpool, PO Box 149, L69 3BX, UK*).

CONTENTS

Chapter Five
DEVELOPMENT AND STANDARDISATION OF
THE KNOWLEDGE QUESTIONNAIRE

Chapter Six
MEASURES OF HANDWASHING BEHAVIOUR

Chapter Ten
THE CONTRIBUTION OF PSYCHOLOGY IN
THE CONTROL OF HOSPITAL INFECTIONS:
SUMMARY AND CONCLUDING THOUGHTS

ACKNOWLEDGEMENTS

Professor G.A.J. Ayliffe, Hospital Infection Research Laboratory, Dudley Road Hospital, Birmingham, for his overall guidance and specific advice on the handwashing promotional materials.

Miss Andrea M. Buckles, Infection Control Nurse, University Royal Liverpool Hospital, for her advice, opinions and unreserved support during the design and implementation of the educational and promotional campaigns in the Liverpool (Experimental) hospital.

Mrs. Mary Cregg and Mrs Carol J. King for the preparation of the Tables and Appendices.

Mrs. Renee Forster, Medical Artist, department of Medical Illustration, Liverpool University, for creating the handwashing promotional posters.

[†]**Mr. D. James** , Technician, department of Medical Microbiology, University Royal Liverpool Hospital, for installing electric handwash counters on soap dispensers.

Mr. C.A. Mackintosh, Principal Scientist, department of Medical Microbiology, Wirral Hospital NHS Trust, for advising on the revision of the experimental data and text. Mr. C.A. Mackintosh was also responsible for the proof-reading and typographical design of this monograph.

Mr. D.G. Phillips of Amoa Ltd., Burbage, Leicestershire, for his technical expertise and involvement during the development of the 'optimal' hospital soap.

Mr C.M. Neads, of the Central Television and Photographic Service of the University of Liverpool, for directing and producing the handwashing training video tape.

Professor M. Twyman and his undergraduates, department of Typography & Graphic Communications, University of Reading, for researching the materials for the educational campaign and designing their presentation for clarity and maximum psychological impact.

Professor J.D. Williams, department of Medical Microbiology, London Hospital Medical College, for administering the baseline, post-educational campaign and post-promotional campaign measurements in the London (Control) hospital, also for his advice on the handwashing promotional materials.

Chapter One

THE NATURE AND EXTENT OF HOSPITAL-ACQUIRED (NOSOCOMIAL) INFECTIONS

1.1 Introduction

In recent times, the general public has come to believe that illnesses are best dealt with by doctors and that the best place to be, when ill, is in hospital. One aspect of such a belief is the illusion that modern hospitals are a safe haven from disease. One might logically anticipate a low risk of contracting a new disease whilst in such an apparently safe environment as a hospital ward. Nothing could be further from the truth! The modern hospital environment and the ever more sophisticated medical procedures can be potent health hazards. When Florence Nightingale said 'it may seem a strange principle to enunciate as the very first requirement in a hospital that it should do the sick no harm', hospital-acquired infections (HAI) were the most feared. More than a century later, they still harm patients.

Infections can be acquired from a variety of sources. By convention, a distinction is made between the community and the hospital environment, as the source of infection. The former are known as community-acquired infections (CAI); the latter are normally referred to as hospital-acquired (HAI), or nosocomial infections. From a different perspective, if an infection is caused by micro-organisms originating outside the body, as from other human beings, animals, or the inanimate environment, such an infection is termed exogenous. If, on the other hand, an infection is thought to be caused by micro-organisms living within one's own body, it is referred to as an endogenous (self-, auto-) infection. Cross-infection implies an exogenous source within the community or hospitals. Not all

HAI infections are preventable. However, we believe that a significant proportion are. Although in our studies we have deliberately focused on HAI, many of the underlying principles discussed here also apply in the genesis of infections in the community at large.

This book describes a new approach to the perennial problem of preventable, hospital-acquired infections. Whilst HAI have been traditionally dealt with by specialists in infectious diseases, epidemiology, nursing, health economics and - not least- microbiology, psychologists were conspicuous by their absence from this exciting and challenging arena. We believe this is the first major attempt to introduce an overriding psychological perspective to the effective prevention of hospital sepsis.

Readers may be interested to learn exactly how the whole affair started. In 1983 the infection control consultant of a major English University hospital (the first author), approached the clinical psychologist in the adjacent University (the last author) and enlisted his help. The reason for this approach was his conviction that the single most important factor in combatting HAI lay in the human dynamics of health care staff. In briefing the psychologists on the basic problem of HAI and its historical background, a very expansive corpus of knowledge had to be summarised. In the rest of this chapter the briefing that was originally given to the psychologists is presented. Readers interested in a more detailed exposition of the subject of control and prevention of nosocomial infections may refer to a number of specialist textbooks [e.g. Ayliffe, Collins & Taylor, 1982; Ayliffe et al., 1992; Wenzel, 1993].

1.2 A brief history of attempts to prevent hospital infections

During the plague of the early 18th century, the policy was to remove the patient, who was considered to be the source of infection, to a field where he / she would either recover or die. Those who cared for the patient were then physically isolated for 10 days. It was believed that foul air caused the spread of plague; physicians wore helmets, long robes and gauntlets and protected their faces with large glasses and a respirator resembling a long beak, filled with aromatic herbs (Dubay & Grubb, 1978).

In the mid-1800s the risk of post-operative infection in hospitals was very high; JY Simpson observed that a man lying on an operating table was exposed to a greater risk of death than was an English soldier on the battlefield at Waterloo (Major, 1954). He collected data on 2,000 amputees who had been hospitalised during and after surgery and on a further 2,000 who had remained at home. He found a higher mortality rate for those who remained in the hospital and called this phenomenon 'hospitalism' to suggest that something related to hospital care conferred a particular risk on patients.

Oliver Holmes, in his treatise 'On the contagiousness of puerperal fever' (1936), suggested that doctors transferred the fever from one patient to another. However this accusation was ignored by his colleagues. The role of the hands in the transmission of infection was convincingly demonstrated before it was known that micro-organisms existed. In 1847 Ignaz P. Semmelweis noted that 11.5% of the 4,010 women admitted to one clinic at the Vienna Maternity Hospital died of puerperal fever while, in another clinic, where all deliveries were carried out by midwives, the mortality rate was only 2.7% (Ackerknecht, 1982). Semmelweis concluded (after the professor of forensic medicine had died from sepsis, which developed when his arm was wounded by a student during a post-mortem on a victim of puerperal fever) that puerperal sepsis in the first clinic was produced by contact with the contaminated hands of doctors and medical students from the autopsy room. He demonstrated the validity of this conclusion by introducing handwashing with a chlorine solution before manual examination. The result was a dramatic reduction in puerperal mortality to around 1%. Tragically, Semmelweis too was ridiculed and was finally dismissed from the clinic in 1865. He died at the age of 47 from sepsis in an insane asylum in Vienna.

Over 130 years ago, in 1859, at the Liverpool meeting of the National Association for the Promotion of Social Sciences, Florence Nightingale cited four major criticisms of hospitals: first, the accumulation of large numbers of sick people under one roof; second, inadequate space; third, lack of ventilation; and, fourth, inadequate light (Walker, 1963). This was well before the role of micro-organisms in the causation of disease had been established. Although Florence Nightingale did not believe in the 'germ theory' of the time, her practical recommendations would have contributed significantly to the prevention of HAI. In the previous year Pasteur had demonstrated that fermentation required the presence of minute organisms, but it was not until 1864 that he was able to prove that such organisms were present in the atmosphere.

In 1867 Lister, who believed that particles in the air caused sepsis, introduced antiseptic surgery, which later evolved into aseptic surgery. Antiseptic surgery relies on the destruction of germs in wounds by the use of chemicals. In such procedures everything that comes in to contact with the wound, or the patient's skin, has been previously freed of germs. Lister used a spray of carbolic acid in his practice. The improvement he thus achieved is documented in his audit of amputations, as shown in Table 1.1 (Goldman, 1987).

Table 1.1   Lister's mortality statistics for amputees before and after the introduction of an antiseptic method

Period	Cases	Recovered	Died	Case Mortality %
Without antisepsis 1864-66	35	19	16	45.7%
With antisepsis 1867-70	40	34	6	15.0%

(after Singer and Underwood, 1962)

Lister also introduced the practice of heat sterilisation of instruments and dressings. However, even the infection-conscious Lister did not fully comprehend the implications of microbial transmission and never washed his hands before an operation (Goldman, 1987).

By the end of the previous century, further advances in clinical bacteriology had been made. In 1890 Halsted wrote that wound infection was, for many surgeons, a thing of the past (Walker, 1963). However, during the First World War, infections caused the deaths of millions of soldiers. Such events were so dramatic that doctors at that time even resorted to the use of maggots to clean dirty wounds and remove necrotic tissue. Much later, in 1935, the introduction of chemotherapy with the sulphonamides raised new hopes for the treatment of infections. After Florey, Chain and associates launched Fleming's penicillin in 1941, an exponential growth in antibiotics occurred (Abraham, 1980; Chain *et al.*, 1940; Fleming, 1929). At the time of drafting this chapter (1993) over 100 different antimicrobials are licensed in the UK alone. Such strengthening of the anti-infective's armamentarium allowed doctors to treat infections effectively and painlessly; indeed countless lives have been, and are being, saved all over the world. In parallel, however, such abundance of antimicrobials has created the illusion that infection, as a 'plague' of humanity, has been forever conquered. The fundamental tenets of infection prevention that Semmelweis and Nightingale pioneered were gradually reduced to a plethora of, by and large, ineffective hygiene-related rituals that cost a lot of money but offer little measurable return, in terms of preventing infections.

In recent years, the long-term, adverse effects of antimicrobials, particularly those brought about by broad spectrum compounds, has highlighted several unpredictable aspects of therapy. Pseudomembranous enterocolitis, for example, is a severe antibiotic-associated intoxication caused by *Clostridium difficile*, an organism that colonises the gut flora, previously disturbed by antibiotics. The treatment, of course, is more antibiotics, though different from the original culprits! Microbial resistance to antibiotics is not a recent phenomenon. What has been recently recognised, however, is the rapid genetic transfer of resistance between different microbial genera. Intestinal aerobic Gramnegative bacilli are particularly susceptible to acquiring resistance to many antibiotics in this manner, some to as many as eight different types, at any time ! Methicillin-resistant *Staphylococcus aureus*, often referred to as 'supergerm' by the Press, is a potent reminder that resistance can, at a stroke, destroy a deeply entrenched faith in antimicrobials. It also compels us to reflect again on the merits of prevention, rather than blinkered cure.

The control of hospital infections has improved substantially from the days when infected patients were left in fields to die. Nevertheless, for every medical advance there is a price. Indeed HAI are inextricably -and proportionately- linked with medical advances, the very factors that seem to predispose to infection in the first instance. Invasive operative techniques, immunosuppressive drugs -and paradoxically- antibiotics and hospitalisation individually and collectively create excellent opportunities for germs, and microbiologists, to thrive. The infection / antibiotic cascade is illustrated in Figure 1.

1.3 The incidence and costs of hospital infections

One in 10 patients in the UK acquires at least one infection whilst in hospital (Ayliffe & Taylor, 1984). In the USA the incidence of HAI has been estimated at 5.7%, affecting over two million patients, at a cost of 2,798,023 thousand US Dollars (1984). Cruse & Foord (1973), in a five year prospective study of 23,649 surgical wounds, highlighted an overall infection rate of 4.75%; sepsis became evident after the patient had left hospital in 13.2% of cases. Elsewhere, patients with a single HAI remained in hospital an average 13.0 days longer than their matched controls and those with two such infections stayed an average of 35.4 days longer (Freeman, Rosner & McGowen, 1979).

In the financial year 1983 / 84, the incidence of hospital- acquired infection in the Royal Liverpool Hospital, England, was 8% (Griffiths *et al.*, 1986). This figure means that, of 25,837 patients treated in that year, approximately 2,067 acquired one or more infections while in hospital. If each of these potentially preventable infections prolonged hospital stay by only one week (an underestimate in practice), the increased length of stay alone resulted in 14,469 (2,067 x 7) 'hospital days' wasted. Since the cost per in-patient day in 1983 / 84 was £ 85.24, the overall expenditure for nosocomial sepsis in that hospital alone accounted for £ 1,233,338, in a single financial year.

Calculating the cost of HAI in monetary terms is a relatively simple exercise. The real cost, however, in terms of ethical concerns, the unnecessary pain and the indignity and disability patients have to suffer, lost working days or even premature death, is far more difficult to evaluate objectively.

Figure 1.1 The infection / antibiotics cascade

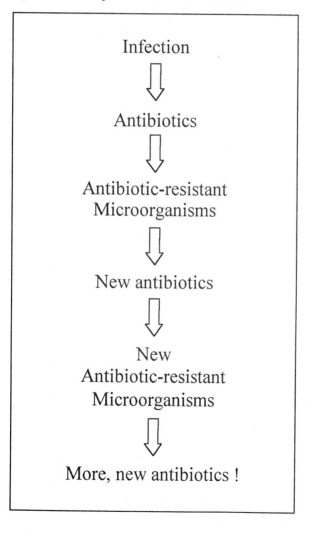

1.4 Factors involved in hospital infections

(a) *The micro-organisms*

In the first part of this century serious nosocomial infections were mainly caused by the genus *Streptococcus*, a group of micro-organisms that produce at least a dozen different tissue-harming toxins and enzymes. Haemolytic streptococci (e.g. *Streptococcus pyogenes*), which before the Second World War were a much feared cause of invasive and rapidly fatal wound infections, today are of relatively small importance as wound pathogens (Ayliffe *et al.*, 1992).

In the 1950s and early 1960s *Staphylococcus aureus*, another prolific toxin-producing organism, prevailed in hospitals; it still does. Hospital epidemics due to penicillin-resistant staphylococci were common in both paediatric and adult wards. The introduction of penicillinase-resistant antibiotics in the 1960s, such as methicillin, led to the decline, but not the elimination, of staphylococcal infections. Staphylococci are still responsible for about half of all HAI, either alone or concomitantly with other pathogens. In 1981 *Staph. aureus*, following the cyclic laws of nature, had re-gained its dominance in HAI. But on this occasion strains emerged that were resistant to all standard antibiotics: one-third of all heart surgery patients at the Royal Melbourne Hospital acquired an infection caused by methicillin-resistant *Staph. aureus* (McDonald, 1982). Epidemics due to this organism have since occurred in most hospitals all over the world. Many patients have died and others are, at the time of writing this book, still succumbing to a common infection against which there is little effective treatment.

Since the early 1960s, intestinal aerobic Gramnegative bacilli surpassed the legendary *Staph. aureus* in the genesis of HAI (Finland, 1970). In the 1970s these organisms accounted for almost two-thirds of all nosocomial infections. In wound infections antibiotic-resistant *Staph. aureus* and various intestinal Gramnegative bacilli are nowadays frequent causes of infection. Different classes of micro-organisms, such as *Candida* spp. and other fungi, are becoming increasingly common in immunocompromised patients (Eickhoff, 1977). Viruses of the Herpes group and the protozoon *Pneumocystis carinii* are often identified in HAI outbreaks (Hewitt & Sanford, 1974). Are all these devastating infections unavoidable?

Though virtually any infection may be acquired by patients (or staff) in hospital, there are certain pathogenic organisms which are particularly associated with hospital sepsis and some which rarely cause infection in other environments. The ability of micro-organisms to cause a HAI depends on their pathogenicity (virulence), on their numbers and on the patient's defences. Patients often have diminished resistance and hence create opportunities for organisms which are, by and large, harmless to healthy people, to injure them further. Such 'opportunistic' organisms (e.g. *Pseudomonas aeruginosa*), usually resistant to most antibiotics, are able to flourish under conditions in which most disease-producing organisms cannot normally multiply (Ayliffe *et al.*, 1992).

(b) *Microbial dissemination*

The major factors in the spread of micro-organisms are the number of organisms shed from a source, their ability to survive after leaving the source, their virulence and the means of reaching a susceptible site (on the same or another person) in sufficient numbers to cause an infection.

Hospital infections can occur via many routes. Air-borne, food and / or water-borne HAI are relatively uncommon amongst in-patients, not because such routes of infection are uncommon *per se:* they are responsible for a substantial proportion of community-acquired infections. These routes however are, or should be, rare in hospitals. Air-borne transmission of the few infections that can be acquired through this route (e.g. tuberculosis) can be readily controlled through the precautions that are normally implemented during 'respiratory type' isolation of infected patients. In the early 1980s the recognition of Legionnaires disease resulted in dramatic improvements in the hygiene of water cooling systems of air conditioning plants. Both hospital and community populations can now be spared from this preventable infection. Water-borne HAI are exceedingly rare in developed countries. The high mortality resulting from outbreaks of food poisoning worldwide, when it reaches the headlines, generates such an outcry that the resulting political pressure is, in itself, an exceedingly effective control measure. Spread by contact remains the principal route of cross-infection in hospitals but, again, the main sources that prevailed only a decade or so ago, such as syringes, needles, medicated solutions, parenteral drugs and even unknowingly contaminated blood transfusions, have all been mercifully eliminated in most countries, through the widespread introduction of disposable supplies and greatly improved sterility assurance in the manufacturing process. Nowadays, it is the hand-mediated infections that account for the majority of literally 'contagious' inter-hospital spread of infection.

(c) Hand-mediated transmission of infection

Price (1938) was the first to divide the bacteria on normal skin into 'transients' and 'residents', a classification still relevant today. Transient bacteria are relatively scarce on clean, unexposed skin. Since such organisms are acquired from extraneous sources, literally 'by hand', there is no limit to the varieties, pathogenic and non-pathogenic, that may be 'in transit' on the skin at any time. Transients lie free on the skin, or are loosely attached by fats, along with dirt. Residents are a relatively stable population, both in size and composition. Any increase in the latter is due mainly to the natural multiplication of the microflora already present.

Staphylococcus aureus, a major hospital pathogen, colonises the anterior nares in about 20% of healthy individuals. Other body sites, e.g. hands, are inevitably contaminated and the organism is subsequently dispersed in the environment, mainly through shedding of skin scales. *Staph. aureus* survives well on drying and can spread by the airborne route, but in hospitals the opportunities for spread by contact are greater. Effective handwashing is therefore very important in the prevention of the spread of not only *Staph. aureus* but most of the intestinal aerobic Gramnegative bacilli that can cause equally devastating, hand-mediated sepsis to patients (Ayliffe, Collins & Taylor, 1982).

One can mechanically reduce the number of resident skin bacteria by energetic, frictional handwashing with or without added disinfectants; the addition of the latter is a process which actually kills bacterial cells. It is the transient skin micro-organisms, however, that are readily transferred from person-to-person and are a health hazard. The aim of routine handwashing on hospital wards (specifically termed 'hygienic hand disinfection') is to free hands from such dangerous bioburden.

(d) *The host*

The host must be susceptible before the organism is able to cause an infection or disease. The body's resistance may be lowered through any of the following factors (Dubay & Grubb, 1978);

❑ *age*, the very young and the very old;

❑ *drugs*, frequent or continuous use of antibiotics or corticosteroids;

❑ *immunosuppressive drugs*, commonly used in cancer treatments and organ transplantations;

❑ *heavy X-ray irradiation*, which causes a breakdown in the body tissue and depresses the immune response;

❑ *malnutrition*;

❑ *chronic diseases*, e.g. uraemia, diabetes, cancer, leukaemia and

❑ *shock*, a sudden circulation failure that may be associated with overwhelming bacterial infection.

In addition to these general categories, the relative importance of risk factors for HAI, and the complex interactions of these risk factors, vary according to anatomical site. Highly important predisposing factors for certain infections affecting, for example post-operative wounds, include urinary catheterisation, a patients' intrinsic risk (as reflected in the underlying condition and type of surgical procedure), length of pre-operative hospital stay, duration of operation, anatomic location of surgical procedure, previous, or concurrent, infection and steroid or immunosuppressive therapy (Hooton *et al.*, 1981).

The medical advances of the last 30 years have played a major role in the characteristics of current nosocomial infections, mainly because of their influence on host defence mechanisms, e.g. the introduction of corticosteroids, invasive diagnostic techniques, ionising radiation, cytotoxic drugs, complex surgical procedures, insertion of prosthetic valves, etc. Furthermore, modern medicine is providing longer life spans for patients with serious underlying disease and thus it is increasing the number of 'compromised hosts'. Such patients are at increased risk of acquiring infection by organisms of relatively reduced virulence, which are normally harmless constituents of the normal microflora (Eickhoff, 1977).

(e) The environment

A wide variety of micro-organisms, including virulent strains, is likely to be in hospitals where many patients, including infectious ones, are aggregated. These microbial populations are also likely to include many antibiotic-resistant bacteria, which can proliferate where antibiotic usage has led to the suppression of previously antibiotic-sensitive populations (Ayliffe et al., 1992).

Micro-organisms can survive on most inanimate surfaces in a hospital ward: floors, walls, ceilings, fixtures and fittings, sinks, blankets, drains, etc.; they are also present in dust and in the air. Ayliffe, Collins & Taylor (1982) summarised the aim of environmental control measures as;

❑ *the provision of an environment that is hostile to the multiplication of pathogens*, e.g. clean, dry, exposed to light with good ventilation;

❑ *the protection of susceptible patients from significant contamination*, e.g. application of dressings and containment isolation;

❑ *increased host resistance*, e.g. through specialist vaccines;

❑ *containment and decontamination of infectious sources*, to prevent cross-infection.

1.5 Infection surveillance and control programmes

As early as 1950, epidemiologists in the Centers for Disease Control (CDC), USA, began to investigate outbreaks of infections in hospitals. In the 1960s more systematic studies were undertaken and better-organised infection control programmes were instituted as a result of these early studies, which highlighted the necessity to establish baseline data in order to assess and control nosocomial outbreaks. Initially these programmes emphasised the importance of surveillance, but in the 1970s they developed further to include prevention and control measures (Palmer, 1984).

The CDC and other agencies have carried out many surveillance and control programmes in the past years, in an attempt to prevent, identify and control effectively such infections. The SENIC Project (Study on the Efficiency of Nosocomial Infection Control) was initiated by the CDC in 1974 (Haley *et al.*, 1980), in order to;

❏ estimate the magnitude of nosocomial infections in USA hospitals;

❏ describe the extent to which hospitals had used an infection surveillance and control programme and

❏ determine to what extent this approach was effective in reducing nosocomial infection risks.

In a representative sample of hospitals they noted that the introduction of infection surveillance and control programmes was strongly associated with reductions in rates of nosocomial urinary tract infection, surgical wound infection, pneumonia and bacteraemia. Essential components of effective programmes included conducting organised surveillance and control activities, establishing an infection control physician, an infection control nurse per 250 beds and a system for reporting infection rates to surgeons. Programmes incorporating these components reduced the infection rates by 32%. However, since few hospitals had effective programmes, only 6% of nosocomial infections were being prevented by universal adoption of this strategy. Amongst hospitals without effective programmes the overall infection rate actually increased by 18%, from 1970 to 1976.

The next chapter will describe the various approaches to the problem of HAI which have been developed in recent times.

Chapter Two
APPROACHES TO THE
CONTROL OF HOSPITAL INFECTION

2.1 Introduction

The previous chapter outlined the various factors involved in, and the problems associated with, hospital-acquired infections (HAI). Many methods have been proposed for the control of HAI which, though not mutually exclusive, can be grouped into three main approaches: *medical, environmental* and *psychological*.

2.2 The medical approach

Before the advent of antibiotics, the prevention of infections relied on basic hygiene, antisepsis, medical skill and common sense. Though antibiotics are now the most rapidly expanding class of drugs world-wide, their increasing use in hospital practice has not appreciably reduced infection rates (McGowen & Finland, 1974). Instead, their adverse effects, not least the escalating cost, has prompted a critical reappraisal of their indication and value (Jackson, 1974; Williams, 1984). Antibiotics can be used to treat, and in some instances, (e.g. contaminated wounds, dental extractions, operations on ischaemic legs, etc.) to prevent HAI. However, they have several limitations: none is totally free from toxicity or short-term adverse effects. For example, of some commonly used antibiotics, ampicillin can cause skin rashes, diarrhoea and vomiting; erythromycin is potentially hepatotoxic (Ayliffe *et al.*, 1992).

However, an increasingly recognised long-term adverse effect of antimicrobial chemotherapy is manifested by an impaired balance of the normal microbial flora. Continuous antibiotic pressure on complex microbial ecosystems can select antibiotic-resistant strains. Even worse, such resistance can be genetically transferred between different microbial families, resulting in unpredictable infections which are difficult, if not impossible to treat. The fact that the frequency of bacterial resistance to an antibiotic varies directly with the extent of its use has been supported by many detailed observations (e.g. Goodier & Parry, 1959). Certain pathogens that are common in hospitals, e.g. *Staphylococcus aureus* and intestinal aerobic Gramnegative bacilli, are primarily responsible for HAI, particularly when antibiotic-resistant. Resistance was first encountered as a major problem in the late 1940s when an increasing proportion of staphylococci from lesions in hospital patients became resistant to penicillin. This was not due to acquired resistance but to the selection of a minority of resistant strains, which were then spread from patient to patient (Barber, 1947). Since many patients who had not received penicillin, as well as hospital staff, acquired these strains, it appeared that penicillin-resistant staphylococci had an enhanced ability to spread and replace sensitive strains. Later investigations by Gould (1958) suggested that the presence of penicillin in the hospital environment may have enhanced the colonisation of patients, who had not been on this antibiotic, with penicillin-resistant strains. It has been estimated that in the mid-1940s the average yearly consumption of penicillin was approximately 375 tons in the USA (Dowling, 1959.)

Outbreaks of hospital-acquired infections with penicillin- and methicillin-resistant *Staph. aureus* are now almost pandemic in the USA (Haley *et al.*, 1982; Thompson & Wenzel, 1982); Eastern Australia (McDonald, 1982) and endemic in several UK hospitals (Bartzokas *et al.*, 1984; Bradley *et al.*, 1985). Epidemics of gentamicin-resistant *Klebsiella aerogenes* (Gordon, 1980; Hart, 1982), an intestinal organism, are another alarming sign of the failure of both control measures and antimicrobial therapy to reduce the incidence of nosocomial infections.

2.3 The environmental approach

The environmental approach to infection control is based on the reduction of pathogenic micro-organisms in the hospital environment. Hospitals harbour both virulent bacteria and infectious people: therefore the potential for cross-infection is virtually unlimited. In recent years much emphasis has been placed on the monitoring and disinfection of the inanimate environment. This approach, relying on continuous microbiological surveillance programmes and staff-instigated procedures, cannot be effectively implemented without substantial increases in laboratory and specialist resources.

Different areas of the hospital pose specific infection hazards. In the operating theatres, for example, there is a special risk of wound infection because of the exposure, often for several hours, of susceptible tissues in the presence of potent endogenous sources of contamination. In the wards patients may be exposed for many weeks to other contaminants from which post-operative wounds will usually be protected physically by surgical dressings (Ayliffe *et al.*, 1992).

Sterilisation, the complete killing of all microorganisms, is not usually necessary (nor feasible!), except for certain items of instruments used for invasive procedures, such as surgical instruments. There are several methods and techniques to measure environmental contamination and to reduce it. Noble & Lidwell (1963) list such techniques for the detection of micro-organisms in the air and inanimate sources. Although the aim of these procedures is to reduce the bioburden, the crude number of bacteria in the air of wards, for example, is not necessarily related to the incidence of sepsis in patients (Shooter, 1965). In recent times there has been a gradual reduction in the number of environmental approaches which were advocated in the early 1960s: through critical revision of old methods and the rejection of those sanctified by tradition, but now proven to be useless or even harmful 'rituals' (Ayliffe, Collins & Taylor, 1982).

Although significant and important advances have been made in the environmental control of infection, over-emphasis of this approach tends to undervalue the importance of personal factors involved in the transmission of infection. It has been known that the publicity given to antibiotics and antiseptic soaps has resulted in less attention by hospital personnel to handwashing, change of clothing, attire in isolation rooms and to other sensible precautions (Altemeier, 1979). It has also been observed that the emphasis on environmental monitoring and other technological approaches in recent years has attenuated in-service training, which would promote behaviours that are likely to reduce infections in the first instance (American Hospital Association, 1974; Haley & Shachtman, 1980).

Studies of staphylococcal and streptococcal infections in nurseries have indicated that, although environmental contamination is common with these pathogens, the major mode of transmission involves direct contact and their control is almost entirely dependent on controlling direct contact. Even in the case of salmonella infections and other intestinal diseases, a large proportion of HAI are not directly food-borne: their transmission involves patient-to-patient or staff-to-patient routes. If the predominant epidemiological pattern in the transmission of HAI involves direct contact between people, as opposed to the acquisition of organisms from the environment, then the success or failure of an infection control programme can be related to the amount of effort being expended in controlling personal contact (Hinton, 1971). Surgical wounds, in particular, are often infected by direct contact in the wards. When infection occurs in this way, it is often the result of poor technique, or a breach of aseptic discipline. The psychological approach is aimed at reducing such staff-mediated transgressions.

2.4 The psychological approach

Hospital infection control programmes have focused more upon technological and engineering approaches than upon influencing the behaviour of hospital personnel. A survey in the European Region of the World Health Organisation reviewed research programmes in hospital infection control. Of the 61 programmes listed, only one centred on social control measures (Wahba, 1977). In the USA increasing emphasis has been placed on social factors, largely due to the Hospital Infections Program of the Centers for Disease Control (CDC). The medical epidemiologists of CDC, as a result of their experience with infection control problems, outlined some basic principles of social influence and developed a scheme that recognised the importance of such factors (Raven, Freeman & Haley, 1982). The psychological approach is based on the animate environment and concentrates on:

i   staff awareness;

ii understanding of infection control and

iii adherence to established preventive practices.

The single most important influence on HAI can only be minimised by changing the attitudes and behaviour of doctors and nurses. Though psychological input in this field has been limited, the potential contribution of psychology in the control of HAI has already been recognised (Bryan & Deever, 1981; Larson, 1983a; Raven & Haley, 1982). The current literature in this field divides into two major recommendations: the need for staff education in infection control and the need to increase staff compliance with infection control measures.

Education and specific training in infection control is necessary if policy recommendations are to be carried out. It has been noted that many physicians are unaware of the basic concepts of infection control and, in most hospitals, nurses are far better informed (Maki, 1978; Raven & Haley, 1982). Although microbiology and immunology are given high priority in medical students' education, the need to assimilate a large amount of academic knowledge (on, for example, pathogenic bacteria, diagnosis and treatment of infectious diseases), allows little time to dwell on the prevention of hospital infections (Sawyer *et al.*, 1978). The four major objectives of training in microbiology and infection are frequently based on an understanding of (Neu, 1978):

❑ cell biology;

❑ basic host-microbe interactions;

❑ relevant medical microbiology and

❑ the principles of antimicrobial therapy.

Neu points out that such emphasis leads to particular ways of dealing with clinical problems, e.g. 'If culture results indicate that the patient is improving, the first law of therapeutics is followed: he's doing well; let's continue the antibiotics'. Many students graduate from medical school using antimicrobial agents as a substitute for diagnostic acumen, without a deep understanding of how diagnostic resources should be properly used. The principles and procedures necessary in the control of HAI must be incorporated into medical school curricula, as a first step in making medical staff aware of the importance of preventing such infections.

A widespread lack of understanding and awareness of infection control is one possible reason for poor adherence to the control measures, the second is compliance. There is difficulty in ensuring compliance from individuals who habitually fail to comply, particularly if they do not understand the importance of compliance. Another fundamental reason for low compliance amongst medical staff is the status and the prestige in which physicians are held. Bromley (1983) and Raven & Haley (1982) noted that staff had certain stereotyped views about themselves and others: physicians often see themselves as above reproach.

The clear status differences between different categories of staff may be responsible for the low compliance of physicians. The importance of their behaviour is evident in a number of ways: they are less likely than other hospital staff to follow infection control policies, they are more resistant to implementing new policies and to adopt corrective action with regard to infection control; they also occasionally instruct nurses to carry out procedures counter to hospital policy (Raven & Haley, 1982). Thus a training programme for physicians should include more tuition in epidemiology and in the factors that tend to increase the risk of HAI: simple techniques of asepsis (e.g. handwashing and correct handling of contaminated articles) should attract greater emphasis. In addition, physicians should be made more aware of their own importance as role models for others (Larson, 1983a; Laufman, 1983). However, as shall be discussed in subsequent chapters, improved education does not necessarily lead to implementation of the acquired knowledge.

The largest descriptive study ever undertaken in this area was the SENIC project - the Study on the Efficacy of Nosocomial Infection Control (Haley *et al.*, 1980;

Raven & Haley, 1982). The specific objectives of the SENIC project included enumerating the different approaches to infection control that have been practised in North America over recent years and determining their effectiveness by an in-depth study in a representative sample of USA hospitals. Of 6500 general hospitals initially approached, a representative sample of 433 was selected for study. A random sample of Infection Control Nurses (ICN) and staff nurses from these hospitals was asked to complete questionnaires and then interviewed in depth. Their perceptions of the problems experienced and the effective methods of influencing staff were elicited and documented.

The following is a description of some of the major findings from the SENIC study. Firstly, staff nurses and ICNs (or equivalent grades) rated 'attending physicians' as being possibly less likely to comply with Isolation Policy requirements than nursing and non-medical staff. Secondly, when presented with scenarios of offending behaviour, nurses reported they were less likely to deal directly with 'attending physician violators' than with 'nursing violators'. On the other hand, physicians reported that they were more likely to deal directly with 'attending physicians violators' than with 'nursing violators'. That is, doctors and nurses were more likely to deal directly with members of their own profession than another. Thirdly, the perceived power of the ICN to influence others was investigated. They were presented with several scenarios and asked how successful they thought they would be in getting various grades of staff to comply. Again, the ICNs thought they would be significantly less successful in influencing physicians than nurses. Fourthly, an attempt was made to explore the perceived methods of social influence that ICNs believe to be effective. Six bases of perceived power were considered:

1 **Coercive power**: is that which stems from the ability of the influencing agent to mediate *punishment* for the target: *Warn the nurse of possible disciplinary action or possible dismissal.*

2 **Reward power**: stems from the ability to mediate rewards: *Point out to the nurse that your evaluations carry some weight; that you might be able to help the nurse in the future.*

3 **Legitimate power**: grows out of the target's acceptance of a role relationship with the agent that obligates the target to comply with the request of the agent: *Emphasise your position as ICN and the nurse's obligation to comply with your recommendation in this matter.*

4 **Referent power**: occurs when the target uses others as a *frame of reference*, as a standard for evaluating his / her behaviour: *Emphasise that other nurses in the hospital follow proper procedures.*

5 **Expert power**: stems from the target's attributing superior knowledge or ability to the agent, i.e. the agent knows best, knows what is correct: *Emphasise your expertise regarding infection control procedures.*

6 **Informational power**: arises from the persuasiveness of the information communicated by the agent to the target: *Indicate the basis for techniques, citing available evidence, hospital data, or journal references, etc..*

Informational power was most frequently selected; expert power was the next most likely to be used. Although ICNs tended to prefer informational power overall, their second most likely choices were expert power with physicians, but referent and legitimate power with nurses. Hinton (1971) stressed the importance of information, particularly that coming from an 'expert', and therefore a respected source. These findings, and others discussed below, were taken into consideration when formulating the educational and promotional campaigns used in our study, e.g. the information given in the educational campaign (Chapter Eight) came from the expert sources of the hospital's Infection Control Doctor and ICN.

A similar kind of descriptive study was subsequently reported by Seto *et al.* (1988), who investigated the 'influencing tactics' employed by Infection Control Nurses. In the first phase of the study a panel of 44 ICNs was asked to study 58 influencing tactics identified by Kipnis, Schmidt & Wilkinson (1980) and to indicate how frequently they used each tactic to influence other nurses. A questionnaire embodying 23 tactics was then constructed and circulated to a sample of 881 nurses. For each of the tactics, which was briefly described, the nurses were asked to indicate whether they would (a) 'willingly comply', (b) 'reluctantly comply', or (c) 'not comply'. They were also asked whether the tactic was 'acceptable to them'.

The twenty-three influencing tactics were collapsed into eight main categories, as follows:

Rationality	⇨	*Use of facts and data*
Ingratiation	⇨	*The creation of goodwill*
Coalition	⇨	*Mobilising other staff*
Bargaining	⇨	*Exchange of benefits or favours*
Upward Appeal	⇨	*Support of higher authorities*
Assertive	⇨	*Direct and forceful approach*
Ignoring	⇨	*Withdrawing attention or co-operation*
Professional	⇨	*Specific guidance on infection control*

Of the above categories, 'rationality' was reported to be the most frequently used by ICNs while 'rationality' and 'professional' were the two tactics with which the nurses reported they would most 'willingly comply'. These two tactics appear very similar to the 'informational power' persuasive technique most frequently endorsed in the SENIC project.

A number of compliance studies have focused on hand hygiene and handwashing practices of hospital staff. In a multi-centre investigation carried out in intensive care units in Denmark and Norway (Zimakoff *et al.*, 1988a), the hand hygiene practices of hospital staff were directly observed. Of 1015 patient procedures carried out by 164 staff in two Danish hospitals, only 40% were followed by handwashing. Similarly, of 594 patient procedures observed in two Norwegian hospitals, only 51% were followed by handwashing. These results are in line with those obtained in an earlier American study (Albert & Condie, 1981). The

Scandinavian team carried out a further large scale study by questionnaire to determine the factors that serve to promote or deter hygienic handwashing practices (Zimakoff *et al.*, 1988b). The most commonly reported interfering factor was the 'detrimental effect on the skin'. This is in line with the earlier study of Larson & Killien (1982), who showed that individuals who handwashed infrequently, less than eight times per day, placed significantly more value on the detrimental effect of frequent handwashing on their own skin (and on the handwashing practices of their own colleagues), than did individuals who washed frequently. The authors concluded that more emphasis should be placed on minimising deterrents, especially any detrimental effects on the skin, and also on the use of peer pressure. These factors have been taken into account in our study during the formulation of a new soap for hospital staff (Chapter Seven) and during the planning of a promotional campaign (Chapter Eight).

2.5 Summary

The three main approaches to the control of HAI have been briefly described in this chapter - medical, environmental and psychological. While the first two have been pursued for many years, the psychological approach is a relatively new approach. Several studies have investigated the methods of social influence used by Infection Control Nurses and self-reported likely compliance of general nurses with such procedures (Raven & Haley, 1982; Seto *et al.*, 1988). There seems to be a consensus so far, that the provision of information is the most influential method. This is in keeping with Ajzen & Fishbein's 'Theory of Reasoned Action' (1980), which assumes that people do consider the implications of their actions before they engage in a given behaviour and suggests that a concerted informational campaign could increase compliance with basic infection control procedures.

In the next chapter we will describe our aims and general theoretical approach to the problem of HAI which form the basis for the work described in subsequent chapters.

Chapter Three

RATIONALE AND DESIGN OF
THE EXPERIMENTAL APPROACH

3.1 Introduction

The aims of the Liverpool study which will be described in this and subsequent chapters were several but included the following:

1 The development of tools for the measurement of staff attitudes towards, and knowledge of, the causes and methods for prevention of hospital-acquired infections (HAI).

2 The application of these tools to establish prevailing knowledge levels and attitudes among medical and nursing staff in two large teaching hospitals. The same data were also to be used as baseline for the evaluation of the effectiveness of subsequent interventions.

3 The development of methods for studying and monitoring one of the crucially-important behaviours in the prevention of HAI, namely the frequency and quality of handwashing amongst medical and nursing staff.

4 The use of these methods to compare actual handwashing practices with those deemed desirable for effective HAI prevention. Once again, these data were also used to provide a baseline for the evaluation of the effects of subsequent interventions.

5 The development of an optimal soap, to remove one of the possible deterrents to frequent handwashing.

6 The implementation and evaluation of an educational campaign, aimed primarily at making relevant information available, intended to increase knowledge, change attitudes and, thereby, change behaviour.

7 The implementation and evaluation of a promotional campaign, designed to encourage / promote better handwashing practices.

3.2 Theoretical underpinnings of the study

At the outset we expected to find, on the basis of some of the studies described in Chapter Two (Albert & Condie, 1981; Zimakoff, Stormark & Larsen, 1988a) and the extensive clinical experience of the first author, that the handwashing behaviour of medical and nursing staff would be far from ideal. We therefore anticipated that the major psychological problem would be how to improve hand hygiene practices amongst these key hospital staff. In considering this problem we opted to use the general model presented in Figure 3.1.

Figure 3.1 Attitude-Behaviour Model

Knowledge ⇌ Attitude ⇌ Motivation ⇌ Behaviour

The theoretical relevance of each of the influencing variables in the Attitude-Behaviour model depicted above, which affect behaviour, is now briefly discussed.

(a) *Knowledge*

Without knowledge of what to do (and why to do it) people cannot be expected to engage in specific infection control / infection prevention behaviours. However, adequate knowledge in itself does not ensure appropriate behaviour. In the general model presented in Figure 3.1 knowledge of the causes and methods of preventing

HAI is viewed as important, only insofar as it affects one of the major components of attitude: namely, the 'knowledge structure that supports the evaluation'.

(b) *Attitude*

The attitude construct has been one of the most influential but, at the same time, one of the most controversial in the field of Social Psychology. The main problem has been the contradictory literature concerning the general relationship between attitudes and behaviour (Chaiken & Stangor, 1987; Cooper & Croyle, 1984; Tesser & Shaffer, 1990). However, in recent years research in this area has focused on the resolution of a more fruitful question, namely the conditions under which attitudes do predict behaviour accurately. This has been accompanied by a redefinition of the attitude construct. One of the most appealing of the recent attempts at definition, and the one we will use here, is that embodied in the Sociocognitive Model of Pratkanis & Greenwald (1989). According to this model, an attitude is represented in memory by three components, namely:

i   an object label and rules for applying that label;

ii an evaluative summary of that object and

iii a knowledge structure supporting that evaluation.

The first of the above refers to the cognitive representation of an attitude, the second to its affective nature (positive or negative) and the third to its knowledge base (accurate, inaccurate, or missing).

(c) *Motivation*

The motivation to engage in a specified behaviour is determined by at least four factors:

i   the presence of a positive attitude to the behaviour;

ii the absence of a negative attitude to the behaviour;

iii the presence of perceived positive consequences of the behaviour and

iv the absence of perceived negative consequences of the behaviour.

Thus, the willingness of an individual to repeat frequently a certain behaviour, such as handwashing, depends on both the appropriate attitudes and the perceived consequences.

The Attitude-Behaviour model depicted in Table 3.1, and the hypothesised influencing variables described above, guided the various parts of the study that will be described in the next section.

3.3 Design of the study

The study was conducted in a number of stages, outlined in Table 3.1, below.

The first stage was the development of appropriate tools for measuring staff attitudes towards, and knowledge of, the causes and prevention of HAI. The investigations which are described in Chapters Four and Five, were conducted in two major teaching hospitals in England. One, subsequently referred to as the Experimental hospital, is an 820-bedded provincial University General Hospital in Liverpool. The other is a London University Hospital, of a similar size and function. In carrying out the attitude / knowledge investigations, care was taken to compare similar professional groups in the two hospitals (e.g. surgeons with surgeons, nurses with nurses, etc.).

The second stage necessitated the development and implementation of methods for studying the frequency and quality of handwashing practices. Because of the nature of these methods, which require the use of special equipment and bacteriological techniques using live cultures, they were restricted to certain clinical areas within the Experimental hospital. These are described in Chapter Six.

The third stage consisted of a series of developments, carried out with volunteer clinical staff and aimed at producing an optimal hospital soap. These investigations were conducted solely in the Experimental Hospital and are described in detail in Chapter Seven.

Table 3.1 Outline of investigations

Stage	Investigation	Chapter
1	Development of attitude and knowledge questionnaires. Measurement of prevailing staff attitudes and knowledge in two major teaching hospitals.	4, 5
2	Development of methods for studying the frequency and quality of handwashing. Measurement of actual *versus* desirable hand hygiene practices and establishment of baseline data in the Experimental hospital	6
3	Involvement of clinical staff, to establish the desirable characteristics of an optimal soap	7
4	Design and implementation of educational and promotional campaigns in the Experimental hospital.	8
5	Evaluation of the effects of the two intervention campaigns on attitudes, knowledge and behaviour.	9

The fourth stage involved the design and implementation of two campaigns to attempt to increase the frequency and quality of handwashing practices in the Experimental hospital. The first, an educational campaign, was designed to influence behaviour through the presentation of information and, thereby, through effecting a change of attitude. The second was a promotional campaign, designed to influence handwashing behaviour directly, by encouraging / promoting hygienic hand disinfection.

The fifth and final stages were an evaluation of the effects on attitudes, knowledge and behaviour of the two intervention campaigns, and also an evaluation of the effects six months after the promotional campaign.

30

The investigations outlined above will be described in greater detail in subsequent chapters.

Chapter Four

DEVELOPMENT AND STANDARDISATION OF THE ATTITUDE QUESTIONNAIRE

4.1 Introduction

This chapter describes the development and standardisation of a questionnaire designed to measure staff attitudes regarding cross-infection.

Preliminary inquiries were carried out in order to ascertain the general areas in which attitudes should be measured. Discussions were held with key clinical informants, including the Liverpool hospital's Infection Control Nurse (ICN), the Director of Nursing and the Senior Nursing Tutor. These consultations led to the delineation of several major areas of importance, for example, staff responsibility for cross-infection and the usefulness of education. Specific questions were also highlighted, including the attitude that *no more can be done to reduce cross-infection* and that *the availability of a broad range of antibiotics is making infection control less important.*

Nursing handbooks and medical textbooks were also consulted to discern the emphasis given to the various areas of infection control (Blackwell & Weir, 1981; Rines & Montag, 1976; Winner, 1978; Wolff, Weitzel & Fuerst, 1979). Relevant journal articles unveiled important areas of inquiry such as the costs and benefits of adhering to infection control procedures (Dixon, 1978; Bromley, 1983; McGowen, 1982).

The exploratory work suggested seven basic components that should be measured.

32

These were:

(1)   the importance of infection control;

(2)   education in infection control;

(3)   the responsibility for cross-infection;

(4)   care of patients with infectious diseases;

(5)   willingness to comply with infection control procedures;

(6)   individual perceptions of the risks of cross-infection and

(7)   staff appraisal of infection control in terms of costs and benefits.

4.2 Attitude scaling method

A Likert scale was chosen, with respondents placing themselves on an attitude continuum for each of, initially, 33 statements, running from *strongly agree* to *agree, uncertain, disagree* and *strongly disagree*. These five positions were scored from 1 to 5, with a high score indicating a favourable attitude. To avoid problems of acquiescent response, 17 of the questions were positively and 16 negatively phrased.

The Likert scale provides precise information about the respondent's degree of agreement or disagreement and it is possible to include items whose content is not obviously related to the attitude in question (Oppenheim, 1979). In addition to the 33-item Likert scale, respondents were asked to indicate which of five reasons they thought were responsible for hospital cross-infection and which for the non-use of hygienic methods.

4.3 Content and wording of the pilot questionnaire

For each of the seven categories identified as relevant and important, at least three questions were constructed to cover different aspects. Respondents were assumed to have the necessary knowledge of infection control procedures, to make the attitude statements meaningful. Questions were phrased in such a way as to relate to the respondent's own experience, for example *the instruction I have been given on infection control has been useful*. General questions were also included, such as *it is not feasible to maintain good hygienic procedures in a large hospital*; this enabled both general and specific attitudes to be represented (Kornhauser & Sheatsley, 1976). Any questions which appeared to have biased content were accompanied by questions to balance the emphasis. For example, the latter question was accompanied by the following statement: *the current infection control procedures in this hospital are effective*.

4.4 Data collection

The questionnaire was handed out directly to the Liverpool hospital staff on the wards by the second author and collected in the same manner. Although this method had the disadvantage that the majority of respondents were nurses, it had several advantages: such as, for example, the purpose of the enquiry could be explained to the respondents individually. The personal contact also ensured a high response rate (Table 4.1).

Another advantage was that, during the collection of completed questionnaires, it was possible to elicit comments from respondents: these included difficulties with, and criticisms of, particular questions and useful suggestions for improvements.

One hundred and seventy-five questionnaires were distributed, 5 on each of 35 wards; 128 were returned completed, a return rate of 73%. This is a very high return rate for a questionnaire study. Hospital cleaners and porters were reluctant to participate and it was decided to exclude them from the main study.

Table 4.1 *Frequency breakdown of sample completing the pilot attitude* **questionnaire (N=128)**

Age	N	Sex	N	Occupation	N
18-20	15	Male	11	Doctors	6
21-22	79	Female	115	Microbiologist	1
26-30	22	Not given	2	Nurses	120
31-35	6			Not given	1
36-40	2				
Over 40	2				
Not given	2				

4.5 Statistical methods

The statistical program SPSSX was used on an IBM Liverpool University mainframe computer to analyse the data from the 128 completed questionnaires. Although 13 items were skewed towards the positive end of the scale (i.e. *strongly agree*) examination of the variation indicated that parametric analysis could be applied.

4.6 Revision of the pilot questionnaire

To safeguard against the inclusion of items unrelated to each other in the scale, further statistical analysis was necessary. Factor analysis was chosen as the best method of reaching a meaningful interpretation of the ways in which the variables were related. The technique is based on intercorrelating all the items with one another to abstract one or more factors in common. Factor analysis was used to eliminate unrelated items and to retain items that had high loadings, indicating an influence on the factors being measured. Using SPSSX, a factor analysis was carried out on the 33 variables. Thirteen factors were extracted.

To identify the optimum number of factors which could be extracted before the intrusion of non-common variance, a scree graph was plotted (Figure 4.1).

Figure 4.1 Scree plot of the optimum number of factors in the pilot attitude questionnaire

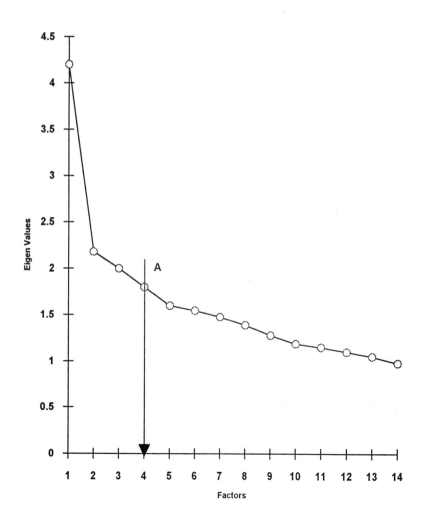

This is a graph of eigenvalues against the factor number (i.e. the order of extraction) and the shape of the resulting curve suggests the best place for the cut-off point (Child, 1976). Considering the scree plot in Figure 4.1 the eigenvalues for the first four factors indicate a curve which develops into a linear relationship at about point A. The point at which the curve straightens out is taken as the maximum number to be extracted, so the first four qualify under this criterion.

Further factor analysis was carried out to investigate the variables produced when two, three and four factors were extracted using both rotated and unrotated analyses. Items which had the highest loadings on the factors were those produced by unrotated extraction of two factors. The arbitrary criterion of 0.30 was used as a cut-off point for significant loadings. Significant items are shown in Table 4.2.

The 20 items found to load on the first two factors included some which were positively skewed, some which were symmetrically distributed and some which were intermediate between those two distributions. This suggests that the factors were not unduly influenced by response set bias but were meaningful. Only 20% of the total variance was accounted for by these items. The remaining random variance was to be expected in an exploratory study of this type which is innovative and therefore unrelated items were anticipated. However the two factors which did emerge were sufficiently meaningful to justify their use.

In order to ascertain which particular attitudes were being measured, *the a priori* category of each item was used (Table 4.2). This showed that factor one was measuring appraisal and willingness to comply, and factor two was measuring the appraisal of infection control. Factor one consisted of the following *a priori* categories: appraisal (4 items), willingness to comply (4), education (1), importance (1), care of patients (1) and individual perceptions (1). Factor two consisted of: appraisal (4 items), education (1), importance (1), individual perceptions (1) and responsibility (1).

Table 4.2 Content and a priori categories for the pilot attitude questionnaire items

Item	Loading	Question	*a priori* category
Factor one			
22	0.620	Little can be done to further reduce cross-infection	Appraisal
7	0.597	Hygiene courses are only necessary for specialists, not all medical staff	Willingness to comply
4	0.569	Specific hospital training in infection control is important	Education
19	0.553	All doctors / nurses should attend occasional refresher courses to maintain standards	Willingness to comply
21	0.547	Even if all hospital staff observed the correct procedures whenever necessary, cross-infection would not be significantly reduced	Appraisal
1	0.508	Infection control procedures should be given a high priority	Importance
20	0.501	Continued assessment and change would be useful in the control of infection	Appraisal
27	0.490	It is not possible to maintain good hygiene procedures in a large hospital	Appraisal
12	0.482	Patients have a right to high hygiene standards even if the staff must spend more time on each procedure	Care of patients
24	0.432	Hospital-acquired infections cause only minor illnesses	Individual perception

(continued)

Item	Loading	Question	*a priori* category
Factor one			
14	0.421	If a doctor / nurse suspects a colleague of an unhygienic practice he / she should explain it to them	Willingness to comply
17	0.402	It is necessary for doctors / nurses to read current journals relevant to their work	Willingness to comply
Factor two			
6	0.520	The instruction given on infection control is useful	Education
2	0.502	Now that antibiotics are more readily available, preventative measures are less important	Importance
23	0.405	Hospital patients are very susceptible to cross-infection	Individual perception
31	0.370	Constant handwashing, use of aseptic techniques, etc. is bad for the hands	Appraisal
30	0.316	There is not enough time to adhere to infection control procedures	Appraisal
8	0.311	The ward sister should be held solely responsible for any cross-infection which occurs on her ward	Responsibility
29	0.301	The current infection control procedures are effective	Appraisal
3	0.300	Total hygiene is a luxury which the busy nurse / doctor can seldom afford	Appraisal

Of the original 33, the 20 items remaining after the factor analysis were reviewed using the comments and suggestions made by staff who had completed the questionnaires. Some of the items were reworded, clarified or simplified: for example, *total hygiene* was not fully understood and was altered to *strict adherence to control of infection procedures.*

The item *Infection control procedures should be given a high priority* was felt to be too general and a separate questionnaire was designed to investigate this area. *Specific hospital training in infection control is important* was often answered by nurses *strongly agree - for doctors only.* This item was therefore split into two questions to allow occupation to be considered, namely *more training in infection control is needed for nursing staff* and *more training in infection control is needed for medical staff.* Respondents were also asked to state whether they had received training in infection control. The final questionnaire is presented in Appendix A.

4.7 Validation / baseline samples

The attitude questionnaire was distributed in both the Liverpool (Experimental) and the London (Control) hospitals, in order to assess the attitudes of medical and nursing staff towards HAI and to establish a baseline against which the effects of future interventions in the Experimental hospital could be evaluated.

(a) *Medical staff*

Doctors in both hospitals received the attitude questionnaire by internal mail, together with an explanatory letter. Five hundred doctors were chosen randomly from each hospital using the medical staff lists; consultants, senior registrars, registrars, senior house officers and house officers, were all included. Seventy-six doctors from the Experimental hospital completed the attitude questionnaire giving a return rate of 15% and 38 from the Control hospital, a return rate of 8%.

(b) *Nursing staff*

Nurses were asked to complete the questionnaires at the end of lectures in the nursing colleges at both the Experimental and the Control hospitals. All nurses were at second or third year level and had acquired practical ward experience. This method of distribution produced high return rates. Of 125 attitude questionnaires, given out in each college, 103 were completed in the Experimental hospital (82%) and 122 in the Control hospital (98%). A breakdown of the validation samples is given in Table 4.3. This shows that the members and grades of staff participating in the two hospitals were sufficiently similar to enable comparisons to be drawn.

4.8 Results

(a) *Mean differences between hospital samples*

For each of the 20 questions of the attitude questionnaire, means and standard deviations were calculated for the two hospital samples separately. To assess whether there was a real difference in staff responses between the hospitals, t-test and significance levels were computed for each question. At the 0.05 level of significance for two-tailed tests, t is significant if it is numerically greater than 2.00, for samples of size 60, or more. Four questions produced significantly different responses between the hospitals:

Question 4, *More training in infection control is needed for medical staff,* produced a higher level of endorsement in the Control hospital. This may be explained by the fact that more nurses and fewer doctors were included in this sample. This is supported by the responses to Question 5, *More training in infection control is needed for nursing staff,* with the Control hospital sample showing a lower endorsement rate, although the difference was not statistically significant:

Question 5, *The instruction I have been given on infection control has been useful,* was significantly more frequently endorsed in the Control hospital. This is consistent with the number of respondents who indicated that they had received some training in infection control: 24% in the Liverpool hospital, compared with 66% in the London hospital:

Question 7, *The ward sister should be held principally responsible for any cross-infection which occurs on her ward,* produced significantly higher agreement in the Control hospital. This may be due to a different approach to teaching at the Liverpool hospital, which gives emphasis to collective responsibility, and also to the effect of infections surveillance and information from the Infection Control Nurse. Alternatively, staff at the Liverpool hospital may have had greater first hand experience of infection outbreaks:

Question 20, *Constant handwashing, use of aseptic techniques etc., is bad for the hands,* was endorsed significantly more often in the Experimental than in the Control hospital. This may be due to differences in washing facilities, soap, and other amenities between the two hospitals.

Of the other questions, 10 produced means of between 3.0 and 3.9 at either one or both hospitals. Fourteen had means of over 3.9 at one or both hospitals. Only Question 18, *The current infection control procedures in this hospital are effective,* had a mean which demonstrated a majority disagreement with the statement. This suggests that staff at both hospitals have little confidence in the effectiveness of infection control procedures as practised at that time.

(b) *Data analysis using factor scores*

For each hospital, mean scores, standard deviations and t-tests were computed for the two factors extracted in the analysis of the pilot data. These are shown in Table 4.4. Factor one, *appraisal and willingness to comply,* consisted of questions 3, 4, 6, 8, 9, 10, 11, 12, 13, 14, 16 and 17, the maximum score therefore was 60. Factor two, *appraisal of infection control,* consisted of questions 1, 2, 5, 7, 15, 18, 19 and 20. Questions 5, 7 and 18 had negative loadings on this factor, therefore the optimum score possible was 25.

Table 4.3 Characteristics of the validation sample for the attitude questionnaire (N=357)

Characteristic	Experimental hospital	Control hospital	Total
Sex			
Male	81	29	110
Female	109	125	234
Not given	9	4	13
Occupation			
Surgeons	24	5	29
Physicians	21	15	36
Other doctors	31	18	49
Nurses	103	122	225
Medical Laboratory Scientific Officers	18	0	18
Trained in Infection Control			
Yes	40	96	136
No	126	49	175
Not given	20	26	46
Age			
18-20	67	57	124
21-25	49	50	99
26-30	15	26	41
31-35	13	9	22
36-40	6	11	17
41-50	15	6	21
Over 50	14	12	26
Not given	3	6	9

43

Table 4.4 Mean scores and t-tests on the attitude questionnaire factors, in the two hospitals

Factor	Hospital	N	Mean	s.d.	t value	P value *
One	Experimental	181	49.84	4.21	1.02	0.896
	Control	158	0.30	4.17		
Two	Experimental	181	9.63	2.96	1.27	0.114
	Control	158	8.89	2.62		

* Two-tailed probability value

There were no significant differences between the two hospitals' overall scores on factors one and two. The means and standard deviations were calculated for each factor by occupational group in the two hospitals separately. T-tests were computed to test for significant differences. These are shown in Table 4.5.

There was no significant difference between scores on factor one between the physicians or other medical specialists in the two hospitals. However, surgeons in the Experimental hospital had a significantly more positive attitude towards the appraisal of, and willingness to comply with, infection control procedures, than had surgeons in the Control hospital. This may reflect an overall unwillingness to co-operate, as only five surgeons in the Control hospital returned completed questionnaires. Nurses in the London hospital were, by comparison, slightly more positive on this factor than were their counterparts in the Liverpool hospital, but the difference was not statistically significant (Table 4.5, Factor one).

There was no significant difference between scores on factor two between surgeons, other medical specialists or nurses in the two hospitals. However, physicians in the Liverpool hospital were significantly more positive in their attitudes towards the appraisal of infection control procedures, in terms of costs and benefits, than were physicians in the London hospital (Table 4.5, Factor two).

44

Table 4.5 Mean scores and t-tests for factors one and two, by occupational group, in the two hospitals

Occupational group	Hospital	N	Mean	s.d.	t value	P value *
Factor one						
Surgeons	Experimental	24	50.42	4.55	2.35	0.027
	Control	5	45.40	2.97		
Physicians	Experimental	21	50.48	5.19	1.77	0.086
	Control	15	47.60	4.19		
Other Medical Specialists	Experimental	31	50.13	4.54	0.05	0.960
	Control	18	50.10	5.42		
Nurses	Experimental	105	49.50	3.76	0.275	0.786
	Control	120	50.88	3.76		
Factor two						
Surgeons	Experimental	24	10.00	2.65	0.31	0.757
	Control	5	9.60	2.30		
Physicians	Experimental	21	11.05	2.13	2.57	0.015
	Control	15	8.80	3.12		
Other Medical Specialists	Experimental	31	9.06	3.20	1.04	0.302
	Control	18	9.94	2.07		
Nurses	Experimental	105	9.43	3.09	1.87	0.063
	Control	120	8.73	2.63		

* Two-tailed probability value

4.9 Discussion

In general, the results of the attitude questionnaire suggested that both medical and nursing staff displayed a positive attitude to infection control. Few differences between hospitals and occupational groups on these issues studied were apparent. Despite these encouraging findings we still wanted to demonstrate whether we could further enhance positive attitudes towards the prevention of hospital infections.

These baseline results were subsequently used to establish attitude change after the intervention programmes, which were conducted in the Liverpool hospital. These programmes are described in detail in Chapter Eight and the results presented in Chapter Nine.

Chapter Five

DEVELOPMENT AND STANDARDISATION OF THE KNOWLEDGE QUESTIONNAIRE

5.1 Introduction

This chapter describes the development and standardisation of a questionnaire to measure staff knowledge concerning the causes of hospital-acquired infections (HAI) and the appropriate infection control principles.

As with the attitude questionnaire, the advice of key informants was sought. Discussions were held with the Senior Lecturers in Medical Microbiology and the Senior Nursing Tutors at both hospitals. These consultations clarified the areas of knowledge taught in the medical schools and nursing colleges at that time. The five general areas thought to be important in the knowledge of infection control were designated as:

(1) *properties of micro-organisms,*

(2) *transmission of micro-organisms,*

(3) *aseptic and hygienic techniques,*

(4) *general knowledge of cross-infection* and

(5) *infectious diseases.*

General medical and nursing textbooks were consulted to ascertain the type of questions which would be relevant in each section and to check the answers of questions so raised (Benenson, 1975; Collee, 1976; Cruickshank *et al.*, 1973; Emerton, 1976; Fahlberg & Groschel, 1978). Ten questions were devised for each area to be measured.

To measure staff knowledge in the simplest and most direct manner, a series of statements was presented to which the respondent could answer *true*, false or *don't know*. Two marks were awarded for a correct answer, 1 for *don't know* and 0 for an incorrect answer. Thus a total score of 100 was possible.

Because, originally, a total of 50 questions was used, the question length was kept to a minimum, generally of less than 10 words per question. Statements which could only ever be either true or false were used. Statements which may be either true or false, depending on other factors, were avoided; therefore only statements which were proven fact and not open to interpretation were chosen.

The initial distribution of the knowledge questionnaires, and the subjects to whom they were given, was as for the attitude questionnaire (Chapter Four). One hundred and seventy five questionnaires were distributed, of which 124 were completed: a return rate of 70.9%.

5.2 Statistical methods

The frequency of responses to each question was calculated by use of the statistical program SPSSX on an IBM mainframe computer at Liverpool University.

There was a wide range of response frequencies over the 50 questions. Incorrect responses ranged from 1 to 95; *don't know* responses 0 to 74; and correct responses, 20 to 123.

In order to decide which questions were most relevant to the area being assessed, correlations were calculated using the Pearson product-moment correlation coefficient. This describes the degree, or closeness, of any relationship between variables; it has values from 0 (indicating a complete lack of relationship) to +1 for a perfect relationship and -1 for a perfect inverse relationship.

The relationship of each of the ten items in each section with the total score for that section was calculated as a correlation coefficient, using SPSSX. The items with the highest correlations were retained. This internal consistency method of item-analysis was carried out for each of the five sections of the questionnaire. Using a cut-off point of 0.30, eight items were excluded. The remaining questions were assessed in terms of their level of difficulty. This was achieved by rating each question in terms of the percentage of respondents who answered it correctly. The following results were obtained:

Percentage of respondents answering correctly	Rating ascribed to question	Number of questions rated
< 40%	*Difficult*	10
40 - 80%	*Average*	16
81 - 100%	*Easy*	16

Thus the questions were evenly distributed in terms of easy, average and difficult. Only 10 items were assessed as difficult; this was expected as the questions were chosen to measure the minimum knowledge of staff.

The above questions were reviewed in the light of comments from respondents and further discussion with microbiologists at the two hospitals. Changes included re-wordings such as 'germs' to 'bacteria' and 'tissue damage' to 'presence of pus'. The final version of the 42-item knowledge questionnaire is presented as Appendix B.

5.3 Sample validation

After edition, the revised questionnaire was distributed to staff at the Experimental and Control hospitals. Three hundred and fifty-four were completed. A breakdown of the validation samples is given in Table 5.1.

Table 5.1   Characteristics of the validation sample for the knowledge questionnaire (N=353)

Characteristic	Experimental hospital	Control hospital	Total
Sex			
Male	83	30	113
Female	114	117	231
Not given	4	5	9
Occupation			
Surgeons	24	5	29
Physicians	26	17	43
Other doctors	27	17	44
Nurses	105	113	218
Medical Laboratory Scientific Officers	19	0	19
Age			
18-20	65	52	117
21-25	48	55	103
26-30	14	27	42
31-35	13	10	23
36-40	6	7	13
41-50	15	7	22
Over 50	14	12	26
Not given	3	4	7

The validation sample was used to assess the level of difficulty, by rating each question by the percentage of respondents who answered it correctly. The following distribution was obtained:

Percentage of respondents answering correctly	Rating ascribed to question	Number of questions rated
< 40%	*Difficult*	7
40 - 80%	*Average*	23
81 - 100%	*Easy*	12

As intended, the majority of items were of average difficulty. Only seven items were difficult, as the questionnaire was intended to measure the minimum knowledge.

5.4 Baseline results

Overall, staff in the Experimental hospital answered the general knowledge section less well than their counterparts in the Control hospital. This may reflect differences in teaching curricula. Answers to questions regarding particular infections may depend on an individual's experience with that infection. For example, fewer of the Control hospital sample answered incorrectly the question on pulmonary tuberculosis, perhaps because this particular infection is more common in the East End of London than it is in Liverpool.

A greater percentage of the Experimental hospital sample answered correctly the questions on infectious diseases. Total scores for individuals on the knowledge questionnaire ranged from 41 to 81 out of a possible 84. A t-test was computed on the total scores for each hospital and the results are presented in Table 5.2.

As t was <1.960, there was no significant difference between the two hospitals' total score. This was a useful baseline. A breakdown of total scores for each occupational group were computed using the entire population. These are presented in Tables 5.3 and 5.4.

Table 5.2 Baseline scores, on the knowledge questionnaire, in the two hospitals

Hospital	N	Mean	s.d.	t value	Significance
Experimental	202	62.960	8.400	1.94	N.S.
Control	152	65.125	6.236		

N.S. = not significant

Table 5.3 Mean scores on the knowledge questionnaire, by occupational group

Occupational group	N	Mean	s.d.
Surgeons	29	70.586	4.272
Physicians	43	70.163	5.572
Microbiologists	2	68.000	0.000
Other medical specialists	43	70.047	4.006
Nurses	218	60.592	6.698
Medical Laboratory Scientific Officers	19	69.985	4.520

Analysis of variance was used to test the significance of the differences between the means of the occupational groups. A significant difference was highlighted: though all categories of medical staff had similar knowledge scores to each other, producing means of between 68.0 and 70.58, nursing staff had a significantly lower mean score of 60.59.

53

Table 5.4 Mean scores and t-tests, by occupational group, in the two hospitals

Occupational group	Hospital	N	Mean	s.d.	t value	P value *
Surgeons	Experimental	24	70.33	4.23	0.69	N.S.
	Control	5	71.80	4.76		
Physicians	Experimental	26	69.92	5.85	0.35	N.S.
	Control	17	70.53	5.27		
Other medical specialists	Experimental	28	70.18	3.37	0.39	N.S.
	Control	16	69.99	4.96		
Nurses	Experimental	105	57.63	6.51	6.95	< 0.001
	Control	113	63.35	5.63		

* Two-tailed probability value

Due to a disproportionate under-representation of certain occupational groups (e.g. microbiologists), further analysis included only four categories: surgeons, physicians, other medical specialists and nurses.

54

Mean scores were calculated for each occupational group in both hospitals separately and t-tests were computed in order to assess any differences between staff groups in the two hospitals. In Table 5.4 it is shown that there was no significant difference between the total knowledge scores of any of the medical staff in the two hospitals. However, nurses from the Control hospital scored significantly higher on the knowledge questionnaire than did their counterparts in the Experimental hospital.

5.5 Mean scores on the knowledge sections

The mean scores on each section were calculated for each occupational group in the two hospitals and t-tests computed. These are presented in Tables 5.5 to 5.9.

There were no significant differences between scores on Section 1, the *properties of micro-organisms*, between any of the medical staff in the two hospitals. Nursing staff in the Control hospital scored significantly higher on this section than their colleagues at the Experimental hospital.

There were no significant differences on Section 2 between any of the medical staff's scores in the two hospitals. The Control hospital nurses scored significantly higher than nurses in the Experimental hospital on the *transmission of micro-organisms*.

There were no significant differences between any of the medical staff's knowledge on *aseptic and hygienic techniques*. Nurses at the Control hospital, however, scored significantly higher than their colleagues at the Experimental hospital.

There were no significant differences between scores for surgeons or physicians in the two hospitals on the *infectious diseases* section; nor was there a significant difference between the scores of nurses in the two hospitals on this section of the questionnaire.

55

Table 5.5 Mean scores and t-tests for section 1, 'the properties of microorganisms', by occupational group, in the two hospitals

Occupational group	Hospital	N	Mean	s.d.	t value	P value *
Surgeons	Experimental	24	8.63	1.14	1.07	N.S.
	Control	5	9.20	0.84		
Physicians	Experimental	26	8.62	1.27	0.36	N.S.
		17	8.76	1.44		
Other medical specialists	Experimental	28	8.64	1.37	0.10	N.S.
	Control	16	8.69	1.49		
Nurses	Experimental	105	4.53	1.98	6.85	< 0.001
	Control	113	6.42	2.08		

* Two-tailed probability value

Table 5.6   Mean scores and t-tests for section 2, 'the transmission of microorganisms', by occupational group, in the two hospitals

Occupational group	Hospital	N	Mean	s.d.	t value	P value *
Surgeons	Experimental	24	9.54	1.18	0.60	N.S.
	Control	5	9.20	1.10		
Physicians	Experimental	26	9.19	1.13	0.48	N.S.
	Control	17	9.35	0.99		
Other medical specialists	Experimental	28	9.86	0.53	1.21	N.S.
	Control	16	9.56	1.09		
Nurses	Experimental	105	8.01	1.65	4.70	< 0.001
	Control	113	8.95	1.28		

* Two-tailed probability value

Table 5.7 Mean scores and t-tests for section 3, 'aseptic and hygienic techniques', by occupational group, in the two hospitals

Occupational group	Hospital	N	Mean	s.d.	t value	P value *
Surgeons	Experimental	24	9.92	5.52	0.43	N.S.
	Control	5	9.40	1.82		
Physicians	Experimental	26	9.31	2.19	0.30	N.S.
	Control	17	9.12	1.73		
Other medical specialists	Experimental	28	9.39	1.81	0.72	N.S.
	Control	16	9.00	1.59		
Nurses	Experimental	105	9.62	1.86	2.92	< 0.004
	Control	113	10.36	1.89		

* Two-tailed probability value

58

Table 5.8 Mean scores and t-tests for section 4, 'general knowledge of cross-infection', by occupational group, in the two hospitals

Occupational group	Hospital	N	Mean	s.d.	t value	P value *
Surgeons	Experimental	24	14.88	2.01	0.31	N.S.
	Control	5	15.20	2.78		
Physicians	Experimental	26	15.08	1.57	0.40	N.S.
	Control	17	15.30	1.99		
Other medical specialists	Experimental	28	14.82	1.83	0.12	N.S.
	Control	16	14.72	2.05		
Nurses	Experimental	105	11.95	2.35	4.78	< 0.001
	Control	113	13.40	2.15		

* Two-tailed probability value

Table 5.9   Mean scores and t-tests for section 5, 'infectious diseases', by occupational group, in the two hospitals

Occupational group	Hospital	Number of cases	Mean	s.d.	t value	P value *
Surgeons	Experimental	24	13.63	1.77		
					1.35	N.S.
	Control	5	14.80	1.79		
Physicians	Experimental	26	14.00	1.67		
					1.04	N.S.
	Control	17	14.53	1.59		
Other medical specialists	Experimental	28	13.43	1.55		
					2.33	0.025
	Control	16	14.63	1.78		
Nurses	Experimental	105	9.77	2.24		
					0.60	N.S.
	Control	113	9.96	2.32		

* Two-tailed probability value

Nurses in the Control hospital scored slightly higher than their counterparts in the Experimental hospital in all sections, except that on *infectious diseases*, where no difference was apparent. This section requires specialist knowledge of infectious diseases, as shown by the lower score of the doctors not commonly dealing with such diseases.

These baseline results were subsequently analysed in conjunction with the data collected after the educational and promotional campaigns (Chapter Eight).

5.6 Reasons stated by staff as being responsible for cross-infection and the non-use of hygienic methods

In addition to answering the attitude and knowledge questionnaires, respondents were asked to indicate which of five stated reasons they felt were responsible for hospital cross-infection. These were (1) the patient, (2) hands and clothes of hospital staff, (3) instruments and dressings, (4) food, (5) fomites (e.g. bedpans, blankets, etc.).

They were also asked to indicate which of five reasons they felt were responsible for the non-use of hygienic methods. These were:

(1)   shortage of time;

(2)   poor handwashing facilities (i.e. soap / washbasins);

(3)   confusion over correct procedure;

(4)   not necessary;

(5)   forgetting.

Respondents were free to indicate as many of the reasons as they wished. The frequencies of responses were calculated for the two hospitals by occupational group. These data are presented in Figures 5.1 to 5.4.

Figure 5.1 *Reasons stated by staff in the control hospital as being responsible for cross-infection*

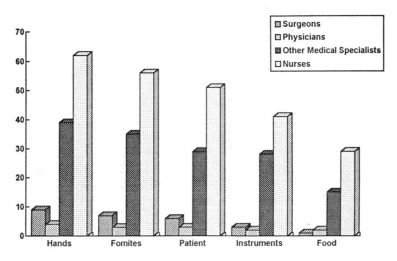

Figure 5.2 *Reasons stated by staff in the experimental hospital as being responsible for cross-infection*

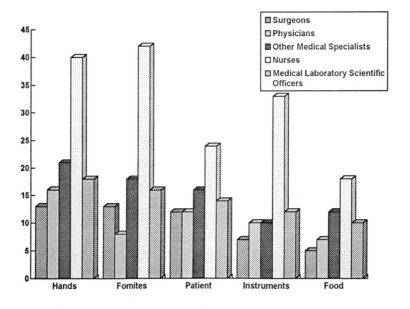

62

Figure 5.3 *Reasons stated by staff in the control hospital as being responsible for the non-use of hygienic methods*

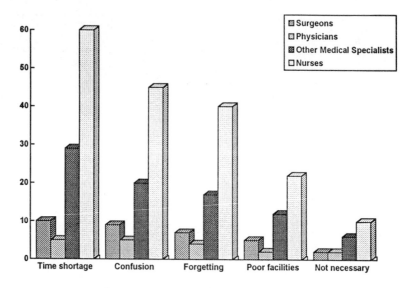

Figure 5.4 *Reasons stated by staff in the experimental hospital as being responsible for the non-use of hygienic methods*

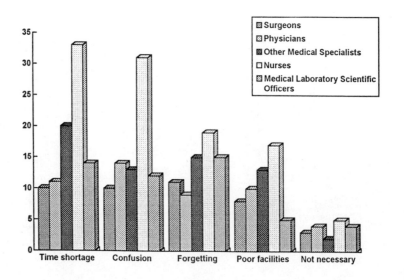

All the occupational groups produced the same order of responsibility and attributed most blame to the hands and clothes of staff for cross-infection.

The same order was produced in both hospitals. There was also general agreement between occupational groups. The results suggest that, among staff, there is a comprehensive awareness of the importance of the hands and clothes in the transmission of infection.

However, when we examined the reasons for non-use of hygienic procedures, the responses of each occupational group in the Control hospital produced the same order: *shortage of time* was the most generally held reason for non-compliance, while *confusion over correct procedures* and *forgetting* were also frequently stated reasons. In the Experimental hospital *shortage of time* was similarly given as the main reason for non-compliance. *Forgetting* was also common as was *confusion over correct procedures*. Thus staff seem to agree in general about why they and their colleagues fail to adopt the correct frequency of hygienic hand disinfection.

5.7 Discussion

The results presented in this chapter establish that the key hospital staff -doctors and nurses- have a high level of knowledge in general about the causes and methods for the prevention of HAI. They are also aware that the major sources of HAI are the staff hands and clothes. Why then do they fail to comply with infection-control procedures? *Shortage of time* and *forgetting* were the most commonly reported reasons. This suggests that the desirable attitudes to handwashing are not 'readily accessible' (Fazio, 1986) and that, as a consequence, automatic processing cannot be relied upon. The latter conclusion is clearly important to the design of effective intervention programmes.

Chapter Six

MEASURES OF HANDWASHING BEHAVIOUR

6.1 Introduction

For over a century, Semmelweis's postulate has remained timely and of increasing significance: handwashing remains the single most important factor in the prevention of HAI. There is a significant association between the frequency of handwashing and the presence of pathogenic micro-organisms on the hands (Larson, 1981). Most hospital-acquired infections (HAI) are hand-mediated (e.g., surgical wound infections, urinary tract infections, antibiotic-resistant-pathogen infections, etc.). Micro-organisms such as *Staphylococcus aureus* and intestinal aerobic Gramnegative bacilli are spread mainly, but not always, by contact transfer (Ayliffe, Collins & Taylor, 1982).

In the past 30 years there has been a dramatic increase in HAI caused by intestinal aerobic Gramnegative bacilli, which parallels the increased use of antibiotics in hospitals and the community at large (Maki, 1978). The problems of antibiotic resistance have been discussed in Chapters One and Two. Evidently, the management of infections by prescribing antibiotics alone cannot be relied on. Mortimer *et al.* (1966) followed the acquisition of staphylococci by infants and nurses from an index infant, known to be a nasal carrier of a bacteriophage-typable strain, whether the baby was touched or not. They were able to demonstrate that the transmission of staphylococcal infections occurs mainly by physical transfer through the hands. A practical technique for monitoring nursery cross-infection was used by Scanlon & Leikkanen (1973) who observed that, two hours after marking one infant with fluorescein dye (a marker, which can be observed by ultraviolet light), the dye could be traced on the hands of all the nurses responsible for the care of the babies. Bacteria can be easily removed from the hands by routine washing; for example, enteric organisms, which were transferred from patients on to the hands of nurses in 90% of cases examined, were reduced by 93% following a short handwash (Sprunt, Redman & Leidy, 1973).

All of the evidence presented indicates that establishing high standards of hygienic hand disinfection - the removal of transient skin contaminants - is the central objective for the prevention of hand-mediated sepsis.

6.2 A longitudinal study of the handwashing frequency of clinical staff during routine patient care

Although handwashing is accepted as the most important health care practice for preventing HAI, few studies have been conducted into its practice in clinical settings. As described in Chapter Three, two recent international studies on handwashing practices in what is undoubtedly one of the most critical medical environments, namely intensive care units, were carried out. In the USA only 41% of patient contacts by hospital staff were followed by handwashing (CDC, 1985). Similar studies by Zimakoff, Stormark & Larsen (1988a) in Denmark and Norway reported frequencies of 40% and 51%, respectively. Clearly, the failure of medical and nursing staff to handwash frequently enough is an international problem.

The aim of our study was to monitor the handwashing frequency of hospital staff, in selected areas of the Experimental hospital, over a period of time. The comparison of the actual frequency with both the ideal and the perceived frequencies, as estimated by hospital staff themselves, was a fundamental objective. This part of the study was also intended to establish the baseline frequency of handwashing, so that any changes in frequency following the intervention campaigns could be accurately assessed.

In order to measure the handwashing frequency in a systematic manner over time, we decided to monitor the use of soap by means of mechanical devices, as described below.

(a) *An automatic monitoring system for the measurement of handwashing frequency*

The main requirements of the handwash monitors were to be simple, accurate and inexpensive. Broughall *et al.* (1984) had previously used a device with three components: a pressure-sensitive mat to register a person standing at the sink, a signal microphone to detect the use of soap and an electronic counting unit to measure the use of paper towels. However, soap usage alone, in our opinion is a useful and accurate indicator of handwashing.

We therefore devised a monitor which, when attached to a liquid soap dispenser, recorded each time the dispenser was used. A five second delay mechanism was incorporated to ensure that one person dispensing several units of soap -a common practice- would only register as one unit. The monitors were battery-operated and therefore did not present any electrical hazard and did not interfere with the hospital's paging equipment. The electronic frequency counters were connected with the soap dispensers via a lead, which allowed the counters to be discreetly hidden from view under the washbasins so that staff would not be reminded that their handwashing behaviour was being recorded.

These modified soap dispensers were installed in two trial areas at the Experimental hospital, a 25-bedded orthopaedic ward and a gynaecological clinic with an average throughput of 60 patients per day. In the orthopaedic ward the monitors were installed under all of the washbasins, in the dirty utility room, clean utility room, treatment room, nurses station, sluice, bathroom, each of five single-bedded rooms and each of four multi-bedded rooms; a total of 15 monitors. In the gynaecological clinic, the monitors were installed under the washbasins in the samples room, the two staff toilets, the two general clinic areas, and one in each of the eight consulting rooms; a total of 13 monitors. Readings were taken every day at the same time and the monitors were also checked for any malfunction. No readings were taken for the initial two weeks to allow the handwashing frequency of staff to stabilise after the unavoidable interest aroused by the installation of the devices. The staff rosters were used to ascertain the number on duty each day in order to calculate the frequency of handwashes per individual staff per shift.

(b) *Baseline data for handwashing frequency*

The baseline frequency data for handwashing on the orthopaedic ward are summarised in Table 6.1. The average handwash frequency per nurse per shift was 5.54.

Table 6.1 Summary of handwashing frequency on an orthopaedic ward, over 21 days

Day	Number of handwashes	Number of nurses	Handwashes per nurse per shift
1	83	13	6.38
2	84	17	4.94
3	78	17	4.59
4	67	16	4.14
5	70	17	4.12
6	100	14	7.13
7	120	15	8.00
8	74	15	4.93
9	61	16	3.81
10	65	15	4.33
11	69	15	4.60
12	69	16	4.31
13	82	15	5.47
14	82	14	5.86
15	97	13	7.46
16	91	14	6.50
17	103	15	6.87
18	99	18	5.50
19	63	15	4.20
20	117	14	7.80
21	85	14	5.31
Total	1759	318	average 5.54 *

* Handwashing frequency was taken to measure that of nursing staff as only two visiting doctors were associated with the ward and their infrequent presence was considered to make little difference to the overall average handwashing frequency recorded on this ward.

The baseline frequency data for handwashing on the gynaecological clinic is summarised in Table 6.2. The average handwash frequency per staff per shift was 7.34.

Table 6.2 *Summary of handwashing frequency in a gynaecological clinic, over 21 days*

Day	Number of handwashes	Number of staff	Handwashes per staff per shift
1	86	10	8.6
2	67	9	7.4
3	50	9	5.6
4	79	10	7.9
5	81	13	6.2
6	97	13	7.5
7	82	10	8.2
8	75	9	8.3
9	53	9	5.9
10	69	11	6.3
11	64	10	6.4
12	67	10	6.7
13	88	9	9.8
14	63	9	7.0
15	90	11	8.2
16	86	10	8.6
17	73	10	7.3
18	64	9	7.1
19	55	9	6.1
20	76	10	7.6
21	73	10	7.3
Total	1538	210	average 7.34

The baseline frequency was very much lower than that which would be expected if staff were following the recommended guidelines, which require handwashing between each patient contact. If the Centers for Disease Control guidelines (1985) had been followed, the frequency of handwashing should be around 20-30 handwashes per staff per shift. The above findings are concordant with those reported by Broughall *et al.* (1984), who noted a handwashing frequency of 5-10 per nurse per shift in a medical ward.

These data provided the baseline, against which those collected following the educational and promotional campaigns were compared.

(c) *Handwashing activity, by location*

It was noticed that some of the washbasins were used far more frequently than others. The handwashing frequency was therefore examined in terms of the washbasins location. The results are shown in Tables 6.3 and 6.4.

Table 6.3 Handwashing activity, by location, on an orthopaedic ward, over 21 days

Location of washbasins	Number of handwashes	Percentage use of washbasins
Nurses' station	481	27.49
Clean Utility room	433	24.74
Multi-bedded rooms (x 3)	194	16.17
Sluice	218	12.46
Dirty utility room	130	7.43
Single-bedded rooms (x 6)	264	2.00
Bathroom	20	1.14
Treatment room	10	0.57

Table 6.4 Handwashing activity, by location, in a gynaecological clinic, over 21 days

Location of washbasins	Number of handwashes	Percentage use of washbasins
Pathology samples room	603	39.20
General consulting area (x 2)	367	12.20
Staff toilets (x 2)	182	10.07
Individual consulting rooms (x 8)	386	3.21

On the orthopaedic ward the most commonly used washbasins were those in the nurses station and in the clean utility room, located opposite the station. These are the sinks which are passed most frequently by staff. They are also areas where staff, when handwashing, are most likely to be seen by their peers and where transgressions (e.g. preparing a syringe without handwashing) would be more likely to be noticed. Conversely, there was very little use of the basins in the single-bedded rooms, though these were often occupied by infectious patients in containment isolation.

In the gynaecological clinic the samples room and the two general consulting areas, which were the most public, were also the locations of frequent handwashing activity. This suggests that social factors (e.g. peer pressure and convenience) may play an important role in determining when and where staff hand wash. Larson (1983a) suggested that an important determinant of staff handwashing behaviour was the practices of their colleagues.

(d) *Self-reports of handwashing frequency*

In order to compare the objective measures of handwashing frequency with the subjective judgements of staff, each member of the nursing staff on the ward and in the clinic was asked, privately, to estimate how often, on average, they handwashed, per shift. Their replies are shown in Tables 6.5 and 6.6.

Table 6.5 Self-reports of handwashing frequency per shift of nursing staff on an orthopaedic ward

Nursing staff grade	Estimated personal handwashing frequency
Sister 1	20
Sister 2	20
Staff nurse 1	15
Staff nurse 2	15 - 20
Staff nurse 3	20
Staff nurse 4	15 - 20
State enrolled nurse 1	10 - 20
State enrolled nurse 2	30
Student nurse 1	10 - 20
Student nurse 2	35
Student nurse 3	10
Average handwashes per nurse per shift	19.5

However, in both clinical areas monitored the personal estimate of handwashing frequency was approximately three times greater than the observed (actual) frequency.

Although staff realise that they should handwash frequently, in practice, they do not handwash as frequently as they think they do. In a similar study nurses estimated that they handwashed a mean of 14.4 times per day (range 4 to 50); there was a small correlation between the stated frequency and that noted during the first month of observations, but not in the second (Larson *et al.*, 1986). Broughall *et al.* (1984) reported a mean claimed handwashing frequency of 24 per shift (range 5-40), with a corresponding actual frequency of 5-10.

Table 6.6 Self-reports of handwashing frequency per shift of clinical staff in a gynaecological clinic

Clinical staff grade	Estimated personal handwashing frequency
Sister	25 - 30
Staff nurse 1	20
Staff nurse 2	10 - 15
Staff nurse 3	20 - 30
State enrolled nurse 1	30
State enrolled nurse 2	30
Consultant 1	30 - 40
Consultant 2	20
Consultant 3	15 - 20
Consultant 4	20 - 30
Consultant 5	30
Average handwashes per clinical staff per shift	24.8

6.3 The importance of handwashing technique in the prevention of hospital-acquired infections

The importance of handwashing as a method of preventing the spread of infection is widely accepted, but the efficiency of the actual technique has been rarely studied. Whilst emphasis is often placed on the bactericidal agent used, it has been suggested that the effectiveness of handwashing may not be dependent on the preparation used but may reflect the physical action of washing (Bartzokas *et al.*, 1983; Mortimer *et al.*, 1966). Lowbury, Lilly & Bull (1964) also noted that the efficacy of method was more important than the washing agent. Sprunt, Redman & Leidy (1973) concluded from their study of the antibacterial efficacy of routine handwashing, that recently acquired organisms are removed from the hands chiefly by the mechanical frictional action of energetic rubbing, rather than killed by a medicated preparation.

In order to study the efficacy of the current handwashing practices in the Experimental hospital a technique described by Taylor (1978) was followed.

(a) *Method*

Twenty nurses, four from each of 5 wards, volunteered. In order to avoid bias, the nurses were not told the purpose of the experiment. They were blindfolded and donned plastic aprons. Five millilitres of a saturated solution of a dye (edicol carmoisine in 70% methanol) were poured into the cupped hands of the subjects, who handrubbed as if they were washing under running water. This particular dye stains red when rubbed onto the skin. The unstained parts of the hands (i.e. those missed by the dye and therefore not washed) were recorded on outline paper hand charts.

This procedure was repeated after the educational and promotional campaigns in the same wards.

(b) *Results*

Sixty-five percent of nurses missed some part of the hand surface; the most commonly missed area was the tips of the fingers. These results are similar to those of Taylor (1978) who pointed out that the implications of inadequate techniques are potentially serious, since the areas most often neglected are those which are most likely to come into contact with patients or contaminated items. The finger tips are also known to harbour more bacteria than other parts of the hands (Hann, 1973; Ojajarvi, Makela & Rantasalo, 1977).

Following the educational campaign the results did not improve significantly from the baseline values. Sixty percent of nurses still missed some area of the hands.

However, after the promotional campaign, which included a video film demonstrating the correct handwashing technique and a leaflet outlining a seven stage technique for effective handwashing, only 35% of the nurses missed some part of the hand surface. Adequate handwashing techniques should be taught as part of the formal training curricula for all staff providing patient care, as this approach appears to be effective.

6.4 Hand carriage of potential pathogens amongst nurses

In order to ascertain the types and density of organisms present on the hands of the nursing staff, random tests were carried out. There are many different hand-sampling methods: the scrub-rinse method (Casewell & Phillips, 1977; Price, 1938), the scraping method (Evans *et al.*, 1950), the impression plate method (Berman & Knight, 1969), the tape-stripping method (Updegraff, 1964) and the swab method (Evans & Stevens, 1976). The technique chosen for our study was a fingertip kneading method, since it is the fingertips that are most likely to acquire and to transmit pathogens. The results obtained by this sampling method were similar with those obtained by the handwashing technique (Ayliffe *et al.*, 1975).

(a) *Method*

Twenty nurses were asked to place their fingers and thumbs simultaneously into two wide-mouth receptacles, containing sterile stripping fluid, and to knead fingers continuously for 30 seconds. The sampling fluids were pooled, poured onto agar plates and incubated at 37°C for 24 hours. All isolates were enumerated and bacteriologically identified.

(b) *Results*

The normal skin microflora consists mainly of *Staphylococcus epidermidis* (*albus*), a skin commensal. An acceptable count from such sampling is considered to be <100 / ml (Ayliffe, Collins & Taylor, 1982). However, of the 20 nurses tested, less than half had an acceptable level of normal flora on their digital pulps. The remainder showed high counts of normal flora, indicating infrequent handwashing. Furthermore, many carried strict pathogens, i.e. *Staphylococcus aureus* and opportunistic pathogens such as intestinal aerobic Gramnegative bacilli; the latter being typical constituents of human faeces.

(c) *Predicted versus actual pathogens present on the hands*

A further 28 nurses were interviewed during routine 'clean' nursing activities (e.g. bed making) and asked to predict what pathogenic organisms, if any, they thought may be present on their hands. Immediately after, hands were sampled as previously described. Only 9 of the 28 nurses had made correct predictions. Well over half did expect some pathogenic organism to be present; half did, in fact, carry potential pathogens on their hands. But though many anticipated that their hands may have been contaminated, they still carried on with various 'clean' nursing activities regardless. This alarming finding is similar to that reported by Moore & Abbot (1980). They realised that attempts to improve handwashing performance by means of displaying to staff a visual growth of organisms from their own hand cultures failed to have an impact on handwashing frequency. In other words, even when documented carriage of hand-mediated pathogens is 'fed-back' to individuals, staff still fail to handwash.

6.5 Compliance of senior doctors with handwashing recommendations

The Centers for Disease Control (1986) recommend that all hospital staff must handwash between patient contacts. Larson *et al.* (1986) found that nurses handwashed significantly more often than doctors. In a previous study (1983a), Larson reported that an important determinant of handwashing was the behaviour of professional colleagues. Larson observed that handwashing was substantially higher in an experimental group when an attending physician, the 'role model', carefully washed his / her hands between each patient contact, than in a control group in the absence of a 'role model'. To test this possibility, a two-months experiment, observing handwashing practices during clinical ward rounds, was carried out. The handwashing practices of senior doctors in the Experimental hospital were observed to ascertain their compliance with standard recommendations.

(a) *Method*

Senior doctors (NHS consultants) were observed during ward rounds. They were not told that their handwashing practices were the object of special observation. The number of patients consulted and physically examined was also recorded. Several of the ward rounds included instruction of medical students. Observations were repeated after the educational and promotional campaigns.

(b) *Results*

The handwashing frequency of senior doctors was extremely low. In fact, only two handwashes were observed during 21 hours of observation! Neither the educational nor the promotional campaign succeeded in improving doctors' compliance. This was probably due to the reluctance of doctors to watch the training video on handwashing, or to read the educational leaflet. These observations emphasise the necessity of increasing the compliance of doctors with such elementary hygiene practices, perhaps by incorporating them explicitly into the medical school curricula.

6.6 Summary

Contact transfer of micro-organisms on the hands of hospital staff is one of the most important causes of HAI. The handwashing frequency of staff was well below the recommended level: only between 5 and 7 handwashes per staff per shift. Staff were more likely to handwash in public areas than in private rooms, suggesting that social as well as hygienic considerations are important in determining behaviour.

Self-reports of handwashing frequency were approximately three times higher than the actual level, suggesting that staff realised the importance of frequent handwashing.

When staff did handwash, their technique was poor: they consistently missed the most important areas, in terms of transfer of micro-organisms, the digital pulps. Handwashing technique was improved by the promotional campaign but not by the educational campaign. Many nurses were hand carriers of potential pathogens. There was no relationship between actual and predicted carriage, although most thought they would have some pathogenic bacteria on their hands. Senior doctors, important 'role models' for other clinical staff, showed almost no compliance with handwashing recommendations. They improved neither after the educational nor after the promotional campaigns.

Chapter Seven

THE FORMULATION AND APPRAISAL OF AN OPTIMAL HOSPITAL SOAP

7.1 Introduction

In Chapter Three we briefly discussed our theoretical model for approaching the problem of hospital-acquired infections (HAI) from the psychological perspective. We suggested that motivation is best construed as a mixture of positive and negative incentives. The latter include any obvious disadvantages for staff that may come about from frequent handwashing. This chapter is concerned with an attempt to minimise one potential negative consequence of regular and effective handwashing.

Compliance with infection prevention measures cannot be achieved without minimising the deterrents to handwashing. Responses to Question 20, on the attitude questionnaire, indicated that many felt that frequent handwashing and the *use of aseptic techniques* was *bad for the hands*. Dry skin, harsh and unpleasant soap and poor washing facilities were often mentioned by staff in connection with infrequent handwashing. Ojajarvi (1981) stressed that 'differences found in the acceptability of soaps imply that for use in hospital the choice of a soap acceptable to nursing staff is important in promoting proper hand hygiene'.

A study of factors for and against handwashing in a USA University Hospital demonstrated that whether or not individuals handwashed frequently, they placed the same weight on reasons for handwashing (Larson & Killien, 1982). Those however, who were infrequent handwashers, placed significantly more emphasis on reasons against, such as adverse skin effects. The researchers concluded that more stress should be placed on minimising deterrents rather than on emphasising the importance of handwashing. Staff preferences were therefore sought in order to establish the most acceptable formulation in terms of colour, fragrance and composition for an optimal hospital soap.

7.2 Volunteers

The subjects used in the colour and fragrance preference trials were volunteer staff from the Experimental hospital. The sample comprised 20 nurses and 10 doctors: 11 men and 19 women. The trials were held in a staff common room.

7.3 Colour preference

(a) Method

Twelve standard colours were removed from a pigment colour chart and affixed onto a demonstration card. The colours included both light and dark tones of yellow, red, blue, green, orange and brown. Subjects were shown the colour card and asked to choose the three colours they thought most preferable for a hospital soap[1].

(b) Results

Individual staff's colour preferences for a hospital soap are summarised in Table 7.1.

---

[1] The word soap implies a hand cleanser, often a solid bar, that is based on natural ingredients. If a hand cleanser is synthetic, it is normally referred to as a synthetic detergent (syndet). Although in this study we specify the composition of the various formulations of liquid soaps developed and tested, the word soap is used throughout this monograph to denote a liquid hand cleanser, whether of natural, synthetic, or mixed composition.

Table 7.1 Preference of clinical staff for a soap colour (N=30)

Colour	Percentage
ST 1 / 25 Red FGR	70.00 *
ST 1 / 25 Green GG30	53.34
ST 1 / 25 Blue B2G	50.00
ST 1 / 25 Yellow NCG	50.00
ST 1 / 25 Yellow HRD	46.67
ST 1 / 25 Oxide Red B30	26.67
Yellow NCG	3.33
Blue B2G	0.00
Green GG 30	0.00
Oxide Red B30	0.00
Red FGR	0.00
Yellow HRO	0.00

* Most preferred

A light red colour (ST 1 / 25 Red FGR), was chosen by 70% of subjects, making it the most significantly preferred colour.

7.4 Fragrance preference

(a) *Method*

In order to ascertain the most widely acceptable fragrance for a hospital soap, 11 popular fragrances were tested. These were placed in 6oz. glass wide-mouth bottles which were labelled 1 to 11. The assessment was double-blind: neither the tester nor the subjects knew what the fragrances were. As the concentration and volume of test fragrances have been shown to be important variables (Wenzel, 1948), equal strengths and quantities of each fragrance were used to ensure consistency.

The bottles were placed on a table and grouped together in random order. The Moncrieff method (1966) for odour preference testing was applied, as follows:

i Each subject was shown how to smell the fragrances: a bottle was picked up, the stopper removed and the subject sniffed it for a few seconds. The subject placed the bottles into one of two groups, 'liked' or 'disliked'.

ii The subject sniffed at the 'liked' group again and placed the one most liked on the extreme left, the one liked second next to it and so on.

iii The subject sniffed at the 'disliked' group again and placed the one disliked most on the extreme right, the one disliked second next to it and so on.

iv This resulted in the bottles being arranged in a line according to the subject's preference. The subject went through the bottles again sniffing at the most 'liked' first and then ensuring that there was a progressive decrease in liking from left to right. This often resulted in reversing the positions of two of the bottles.

v The bottles were randomly regrouped for the next subject.

(b) *Results*

Staffs' preferences for the ideal fragrance of a hospital soap are presented in Table 7.2.

Table 7.2 Mean rankings of preferences of clinical staff for a soap fragrance (N = 30)

Fragrance	Mean rank
Party Time	2.30 *
Wax Fragrance	3.83
Triple Fragrance	3.93
Sun up (lemon)	4.57
Rose Perfume	5.18
Jasmine 1067	6.30
Bouquet 730	6.92
Bouquet P6706	6.97
Deodorant SGB U362A	8.43
Bouquet 572A	8.73
Springtime Dairy	8.83

* Most preferred

A Kendall coefficient of concordance (W) was computed. This is a descriptive measure of the agreement, or concordance, between the subject's rankings. When perfect agreement exists between subjects $W = 1$; when maximum disagreement exists $W = 0$. A highly significant concordance was shown, 'Party Time' being the most consistently preferred fragrance.

As the ratio of women to men in the trial was almost 2:1 it was thought that a peculiarly 'female-appealing' fragrance may have been selected. A further trial was therefore carried out in order to compare preferences for 'Party Time' and another,

84

thought to be a popular 'unisex' fragrance. Fifty medical undergraduate men were asked to smell each fragrance, in a random order, and to indicate which they preferred for a hospital soap. Of 50, 23 preferred the 'unisex' fragrance and 27 preferred 'Party Time'. Therefore 'Party Time' was chosen as the fragrance to scent the final hospital soap preparation.

7.5 Composition preference

(a) *Method*

To assess the relative acceptability of synthetic and natural soaps[1] the frequency of handwashing with each of these compositions was measured using the technique described in Chapter Six. Soap usage was measured in a gynaecological clinic (with an average throughput of 60 patients per day) and an orthopaedic 25-bedded ward. Each trial soap formulation was monitored for 15 days in both areas. The soaps were, as far as possible, indistinguishable in terms of colour, fragrance, texture, etc. The only difference was that of composition.

A standard natural soap was used first in the ward and, in parallel, the synthetic soap used first in the clinic to control for any primacy or recency effects.

(b) *Results*

In both test areas the handwashing frequency was greater during the synthetic soap trial. If handwashing frequency is taken as an indicator of soap acceptability then the synthetic composition was clearly preferred. This finding was supported by the soap preference questionnaire discussed below.

---

[1] Standard natural soap being a pure vegetable soap based product, consisting of a blend of potassium soaps of tall oil and coconut fatty acids, glycerin and anionic detergent (glycerol monostearate): standard synthetic soap consisting of a blend of non-ionic (ethyloxylated alkyl phenol and coconut diethanolamide) and anionic (sulphated fatty alcohol and glycerol monostearate) detergents.

7.6 Soap preference questionnaires

(a) *Method*

At the end of each soap trial, staff working in the trial areas were asked to complete a preference questionnaire to indicate their opinions on the properties of the trial soap and also to indicate the properties that an optimal soap would ideally possess. Nine properties were examined, including strength, viscosity and lubrication.

The questionnaire was scored by comparing each characteristic assigned previously to the trial soaps with those deemed to be ideal characteristics for that property. In terms of 'strength', for example, if the trial soap was indicated to be 'mild', and the ideal soap characteristic was also 'mild', one point would be awarded for that property. If, however, the trial soap was 'strong' then no points would be 'given. One point was awarded if a trial soap's characteristic corresponded to that of the ideal soap. One point was also awarded if the colour was pleasant and another if the fragrance was pleasant.

(b) *Results*

In both test areas staff preferred a synthetic soap, as that was closer to an 'ideal' soap, than was the natural soap. The general hospital soap available at that time was synthetic, thus staff were accustomed to that composition and many complained of 'greasy' hands when using the natural soap.

Considering all the soap trial data, the characteristics for an optimal soap were:

1   colour ST 1 / 25 Red FGR;

2   fragrance F3 ('Party Time');

3   of synthetic composition;

4   should moisturize hands;

5   should be smooth;

6   of neutral viscosity;

7   should lather easily;

8   of neutral lubrication;

9   should be mild;

10   should rinse easily;

These requirements were submitted to a soap manufacturer (Amoa Ltd.), who formulated our hospital-specified soap at a pH near to that of the skin (6.0-6.5). This 'optimal' soap was used in the promotional campaign, described in the next chapter.

Chapter Eight

THE EDUCATIONAL AND PROMOTIONAL CAMPAIGNS

(A) The educational campaign

8.1 Introduction

A review of the infection control literature reveals one overriding consensus: a fundamental need for improved training and education in infection control procedures for the benefit of hospital staff and patients! (Beland & Passos, 1975; Eickhoff, 1977; Gould, 1985; Hewitt & Sanford, 1974; Himmelsbach, 1966; Laufman, 1983; Maki, 1978; Neu, 1978; Raven & Haley, 1982; Sawyer, *et al.*, 1978). Although many authors are convinced of the efficiency of education [e.g. 'expanded efforts to disseminate knowledge of infection control ... would have considerable immediate benefits' (Maki, 1978)], little has been done to verify this assumption. Feldman (1969) states that the nursing performance (e.g. during containment isolation of infectious patients) did benefit from a programmed instruction in asepsis. However, Gould (1985) concluded that many nurses are unable to relate theoretical knowledge of infectious diseases to practical 'barrier nursing'.

In Chapter Two we described two studies of the social influence methods that Infection Control Nurses (ICN) thought were most helpful in their work. The preferred methods were termed 'expert power' and 'rationality' and referred to the perceived value of providing expert knowledge to clinical staff. The explicit assumption underlying this common perception by the ICNs, was therefore in keeping with Ajzen & Fishbein's (1980) theory of reasoned action. That is, ICNs seemed to view staff as highly committed individuals, who will consider the implications of their actions before they engage in any given behaviour. It follows, therefore, that a campaign devised specifically to convey relevant and important information, concerning the principles and practice of infection control, should be effective with well-motivated staff and should lead to, not only a change in knowledge and attitudes, but also changes in motivation and behaviour. Hence the first intervention we attempted was an educational (informational) campaign.

On the basis of the current state of Cognitive Psychology we recognise that for any educational / informational intervention to be effective, the message presented must be processed at various levels and that the greater the depth of information processing, the greater the likelihood of permanent attitude and behaviour change. The educational / informational intervention in the Experimental hospital was therefore specifically designed to impart:

i   theoretical knowledge of infections and their control and

ii   specific information concerning practical applications;

in order to encourage the transition from theoretical knowledge to correct hygienic practice.

The nature and content of the educational campaign are described in the next section.

8.2 The educational campaign materials

(a) *Primary campaign materials*

The design of all primary campaign materials was undertaken by undergraduates in the department of Typography & Graphic Communications, Reading University. Clarity of presentation and maximum psychological impact were fundamental prerequisites of their briefing. (C.A. Bartzokas & M. Twyman, unpublished data).

Three sets of large wall posters were produced, which clearly outlined the Experimental hospital's policies on:

(a) **antisepsis for patients and staff,** which covered skin disinfection, pre-operative skin preparation and shaving, urinary catheter-related infection, oral hygiene, tracheostomy site maintenance, wounds, hand disinfection and catheter care (printed green on a white background, size A2);

(b) **disinfection for equipment in general wards,** which detailed alphabetically the necessary procedures for all medical equipment from 'ambulift' hoists to 'wedges' for orthopaedic use (printed brown on a white background, size A1) and,

(c) **isolation of infectious patients,** which detailed alphabetically the important features of, and the necessary precautions for, all infectious diseases from AIDS to Yellow Fever (printed blue on a white background, size A1).

These 3 posters were affixed on every ward and out-patient clinic in the Experimental hospital, in areas where they would be directly accessible to both medical and nursing staff, e.g. the nurses stations and main ward corridors.

(b) *Accessory materials to the isolation policy*

In addition to the poster (c) on the isolation of infectious patients, a A4-size book was produced, offering detailed guidance on the containment of communicable diseases, the principles of isolation and the appropriate nursing procedures. This book was distributed to every ward and clinic. An abridged A6-size edition was also produced and circulated to every doctor registered in the Experimental hospital.

A series of A4-size door notices, outlining a summary of the essential precautions for staff nursing patients 'in isolation' was also produced. These were printed in yellow and black (warning colours) and were headed Important. One two-part set was created for protective isolation and another for containment (contact / respiratory) isolation. One part was designed to be affixed to external side of the door of the isolation rooms and consisted of instructions such as 'Wear gloves',

'Wear apron', etc.; the other part, designed to be affixed to the internal door side, detailed the precautions necessary before leaving the isolation room, e.g. 'Keep face mask on until outside room', 'Dispose of clinical and domestic waste in a yellow bag'. A further notice was created to accompany infectious patients on transit.

All of these materials included the name and telephone extension number of the Infection Control Doctor and Infection Control Nurse, stating their availability to offer any further advice and to answer queries.

Thus all the basic information on infections and their control was made available to the medical and nursing staff. Together, the educational materials provided all the answers, either directly or indirectly, to the 42 questions of the knowledge questionnaire.

8.3 Response to the educational posters

After the three main posters and the isolation door notices had been on display in the hospital for three weeks, a survey of their usage and acceptability was carried out on the wards to ensure that the respondents had been in the areas where the posters were located; and to ensure that they had been involved in situations where the posters would be consulted. A total of 60 staff (30 doctors and 30 nurses) were asked the following question: *Recently, posters about antisepsis, disinfection and isolation have been put up in the hospital; have you seen them?* If they responded affirmatively they were also asked: *Have you referred to them?* If they answered affirmatively they were further asked: *Did you find them useful?* The responses to these questions are given in Table 8.1.

Although only a disappointing third of doctors had seen the posters, half of the nurses asked had seen them; and those who had referred to them reported that they had found the information presented useful.

Table 8.1   Response to the educational posters of staff in the experimental hospital

	Percentage of affirmative responses	
Question	**Doctors**	**Nurses**
1 Have you seen the posters ?	30%	50%
2 Have you referred to them ?	27%	43%
3 Did you find them useful ?	27%	43%

Furthermore, doctors and nurses on duty in wards, where patients were in containment isolation, were asked about the usefulness of the door-affixed instruction notices. All of the 36 nurses and 9 doctors who had referred to these notices had found them useful. This suggests that staff appreciated the simple and direct advice, which acted as a reminder of the correct procedures, rather than the more theoretical information offered in the main posters.

(B) The promotional campaign

8.4 Introduction

The theory of reasoned action of Ajzen and Fishbein (1980) assumes that individuals are strongly motivated to process and respond to relevant information. This may not necessarily be the case for all hospital staff, all the time. It is therefore useful to consider alternative models of attitude change and their implications for intervention.

The Elaboration Likelihood Model (Petty & Cacciopo, 1986) postulates that there are two distinct routes to persuasion. The first or central route operates with well-motivated individuals, who have the ability and willingness to take part in issue-relevant thinking. The nature of the message is of crucial importance in this context. By comparison, the second or peripheral route operates when people are influenced by factors other than the content of the message; for example, by an attractive or prestigious message-source. The peripheral route seems not to require a high level of motivation on the part of the recipient. In essence the central route works by making people think, while the peripheral route works by appealing to peoples' emotions.

Given the likely variability in motivational level among hospital staff we decided to design a second intervention which would seek to motivate staff and to promote handwashing behaviour directly. In designing the promotional campaign we sought to involve both routes to persuasion. Although the Elaboration Likelihood Model (ELM, Petty & Cacciopo, 1986) had not been published in a substantial form at the time of designing our promotional campaign, we instinctively recognised the need to appeal to staff on various levels. According to the ELM, our approach operated through both central and peripheral routes to persuasion: by stimulating issue-relevant thinking and also using various forms of emotional appeal. The details of the promotional campaign will be described in the remainder of this chapter.

The promotional campaign's principal aim was to motivate staff in the Experimental hospital to act upon the information presented during the educational campaign. Although knowledge on infection control did improve (Chapter Nine), neither behaviour nor attitudes were altered by the educational campaign. The promotional campaign was designed to encourage the application of such knowledge. Some information is inevitably imparted during the demonstration of hygienic techniques (e.g. handwashing) and there is also an element of motivation in the giving of information. The two campaigns were not, therefore, mutually exclusive. The complex relationship between knowledge, attitudes and behaviour has been previously discussed (Chapter Two).

The realisation of the importance of motivation in the control of hospital infections is a recent development of the 1980's. It has been asserted that how well the medical and nursing staff are informed and motivated is at least as important as the use of disinfectants in the reduction of HAI (Mildner, Ohgke & Pfefferhorn, 1984). In her review of handwashing issues, Larson (1984) stressed that techniques from the social sciences should be used to tackle the problems of compliance. Although there is now a growing awareness of the usefulness of motivating staff, the emphasis on environmental cultures and other technological approaches in recent years has diverted attention from maintaining in-service training and promoting behaviours that are likely to reduce infections (Haley & Shachtman, 1980). In particular, there have been no attempts to measure the effects of motivation of doctors and nurses towards preventing HAI. Although consistently applied aseptic practices can prevent HAI, there is a lack of motivation for staff to behave correctly, when there is no immediate positive or negative feedback (McLane *et al.*, 1983).

8.5 The promotional campaign materials

(a) *The optimal soap*

To encourage handwashing a soap formulated according to the preferences of clinical staff in the Experimental hospital was introduced. Its development was discussed in Chapter Seven. In order to publicise the introduction of the new soap and to stimulate interest, a competition was organised, open to all staff in the Experimental hospital. The competition required applicants to think of a name for the soap and to design a poster to encourage handwashing. A monetary prize was used as an incentive. Posters advertising the competition were placed in all the clinical areas. Forty entries were examined by a panel of judges, including the infection control specialists, and the winning entries were displayed in the foyer of the hospital. The winning name for the new soap was 'Pearlesque'.

(b) *Handwashing posters*

Posters are a common tool in the field of health education and promotion, but they have not been evaluated often enough (Gatherer *et al.*, 1979). When little time is spent looking at them they have not been demonstrated to be effective (Brown, 1969). However, posters on a variety of health topics, which were displayed in a doctor's surgery and which carried a minimum of wording, were shown to significantly improve the knowledge of the patients who saw them (Clarke *et al.*, 1977). The target of our campaign was also a 'captive audience' and would be exposed to the poster materials for long periods of time.

As the posters were designed to motivate rather than to impart information, the only wording was in the form of slogans.

(i) Investigation of the clarity and psychological impact of handwashing slogans. An investigation of the clarity and psychological impact of the slogans in the promotion of handwashing had been previously conducted (P.D. Slade & C.A. Bartzokas, unpublished data). The aim of that study was to identify slogans which would help to impart the message that handwashing is an important means of preventing cross-infection. The two parameters investigated were:

i   the clarity of a slogan, expressed in terms of how easily an intended recipient understood the message and,

ii the psychological impact of a slogan, expressed in terms of the likelihood that the slogan would influence people's behaviour.

Briefly, a series of handwashing slogans was commissioned from a copy-writer. Nine slogans were created, which were included in a questionnaire administered to a group of 160 first-year medical undergraduates. They were asked to select the four most appealing slogans and rank them for maximum clarity and psychological impact. A second questionnaire was devised to include the four slogans that had the highest composite ranks, plus six further slogans subsequently suggested by the undergraduates. These were then ranked by other medical undergraduates and a sample of the local community.

To determine the extent to which hospital staff would respond to the slogans investigated in the original study, a third questionnaire was developed to ascertain whether the clinical staff at the Experimental hospital thought their handwashing practices would be influenced more or less by each of these slogans. The slogans finally selected, in terms of clarity and psychological impact, were:

Clean hands save lives.

Don't have a patient's death on your hands: wash them now.

Would you like someone's dirty hands on you ?

Scrub that bug.

Save a patient today - wash your hands.

These were incorporated into several colour posters. Nine designs were deemed most appropriate and most effective by a panel of judges, which included the infection control specialists. A set of these posters, printed on A2-size paper were placed in every ward, every clinic and every special unit throughout the Experimental hospital .

(c) *The training video film on handwashing*

A review of the literature concerning health education and promotion suggests that one of the most successful tools is the video film. In one study, for example, a programme employing video tapes, instead of live lectures, was at least as successful in improving knowledge and changing attitudes as the lectures (Rosen, 1970). Video films can certainly improve knowledge as a number of studies have shown. For example, an improvement in the knowledge of sexually-transmitted infections (Alkateeb, Lukeroth & Riggs, 1975) and an improvement in dental knowledge (Legler, Gilmore & Stuart, 1971) have been reported using this method. However the groups whose attitudes are affected may not necessarily be the target ones: in one study, non-smokers' attitudes were changed, but not those of smokers (Spitznagel, 1969). Behaviour changes have also been reported. Films which advocated health checks for heart disease, cancer and tuberculosis resulted in an increased number of people actually seeking such health check-ups (Haefner & Kirscht, 1970). Out of one, two or three repeated showings of a film on heart disease, the third produced the largest number of people going for check-ups (Kirscht, 1973).

96

Therefore we produced a short video film. The script included the reasons for handwashing, recommended indications of when to handwash and when to use alcohol rub, demonstration of a seven-stage handwashing / alcohol rubbing technique and the relative merits of conventional handwashing and alcohol hand-rubbing. The film was recorded in one ward of the Experimental hospital, so that the location would be familiar to the viewers. Senior consultants were used as the actors, including the hospital's general manager and a leading physician, to give authority to the message. The voice-over was performed by a professional broadcaster who had an assertive and influential voice. The film was 6 minutes long and was designed to be shown to busy staff whilst on duty. Ten minutes is the optimum length for televised information (Olson, 1970).

The video film was taken around the hospital in a mobile play-back unit and was shown on each ward to nursing or medical staff who were available. The response from nurses was very high, nearly all of those asked watched the film; doctors appeared less willing to spend time in this manner.

(d) *The educational leaflet on handwashing*

Leaflets intended to elicit some particular behaviour have been shown to have an impact. When pamphlets on contraception were issued to chemist customers, contraceptive sales rose steeply (Bailey, 1974). A leaflet on gum disease caused approximately one-third of the recipients to contact a dentist (Perlitsh, 1974). The issue of a leaflet about breast cancer to patients increased the number of inquiries about breast self-examination (Hill, 1978). Giving precise instructions about what to do is always important. In one study, a booklet giving detailed instructions about how exactly to get an inoculation was much more effective that one which was non-specific (Leventhal, Singer & Jones, 1965). Bryan & Deever (1981) found that a handwashing drill improved compliance with handwashing recommendations.

A summary of the information given in the video film was typographically designed into a leaflet entitled 'A Guide to Handwashing and Hand Disinfection on Hospital Wards'. Leaflets were distributed to each member of staff after the showing of the video film; additional copies were left in the nurses station for any staff who had missed the film.

(e) Publicity

In most publicity campaigns, increased knowledge appears to be a short-term result, seldom more than 6%, for example in the general knowledge of cancer (Paterson & Aitken-Swan, 1958). The use of films can also be problematic and even produce opposite effects. A film about drug addiction, shown to addicts, was enjoyed by them to the extent that they felt it legitimated their addiction (Winnick, 1963): none stopped taking drugs.

In terms of changing behaviour, mass-media campaigns are most effective when the behaviour required is a single action (Gatherer *et al.*, 1979). Repeated campaigns may show a positive result from the first exposure but little further improvement, or even a retrogression from subsequent ones. Farquhar *et al.* (1977), in their study of cardio-vascular disease, point out that the value of a campaign is increased if skills, which would help people to change their behaviour, are taught in parallel.

We decided to attempt to reinforce the simple message of handwashing by involving external publicity. The publicity for this promotional campaign included articles in two local newspapers and television interviews with the first and last authors. This publicity concentrated on the importance of handwashing in the control of hospital cross-infection.

The general design of the study of two interventions in the Experimental hospital, using a comparable hospital as a Control, is shown in Table 8.2.

In the next chapter we will present the results of the two campaigns in the Experimental hospital in terms of changes in knowledge, attitudes and behaviour.

Table 8.2 General design of the experimental study

	Experimental hospital	Control hospital
1	Pilot study	Nil
2	Baseline measurements	Baseline measurements
3	Educational campaign	Nil
4	Post-educational campaign measurements	Parallel measurements
5	Promotional campaign	Nil
6	Post-promotional campaign measurements	Parallel measurements

Chapter Nine

EFFECTS OF THE EDUCATIONAL AND PROMOTIONAL CAMPAIGNS

9.1 Introduction

In order to determine the effectiveness of the educational and the promotional campaigns described in the previous chapter, the various measures outlined in Chapters Four, Five and Six were repeated in the Experimental and the Control hospitals. In this chapter we present the results of comparisons made over time in each hospital and those between hospitals, at each measurement stage.

9.2 Attitude questionnaire

The attitude questionnaire was re-administered to doctors and nurses in both hospitals, following the implementation of the educational and promotional campaigns in the Experimental hospital. The number of medical and nursing staff completing the attitude -and knowledge- questionnaire at each stage are shown in Table 9.1.

It can be seem from Table 9.1 that, while the majority of nurses approached completed the questionnaire, only a small proportion of the doctors did so. The measurement of attitude and attitude change therefore primarily relates to nursing staff.

Table 9.1 *Number and percentage of doctors and nurses completing the attitude and knowledge questionnaires, in the two hospitals*

Questionnaire	Experimental hospital				Control hospital			
	Doctors		Nurses		Doctors		Nurses	
Attitude								
Baseline	76	(15%)	103	(82%)	38	(7%)	122	(90%)
Post-education	42	(8%)	72	(60%)	62	(12%)	90	(75%)
Post-promotion	64	(18%)	84	(84%)	50	(14%)	85	(85%)
Knowledge								
Baseline	78	(16%)	105	(84%)	38	(7%)	113	(84%)
Post-education	43	(9%)	68	(57%)	59	(12%)	86	(71%)
Post promotion	65	(19%)	86	(86%)	45	(13%)	90	(90%)

(a) *Results*

The two factors extracted during analysis of the pilot study data (Chapter Four) were used. Mean scores and an analysis of variance were computed to assess any differences between the baseline, post-educational campaign and post-promotional campaign data, for factor one *appraisal of, and willingness to comply with, infection control procedures*, in the two hospitals. This analysis was also computed for each occupational group for the two hospitals. These data are presented in Tables 9.2 and 9.3.

Table 9.2 Mean scores on factor one, 'appraisal of, and willingness to comply with, infection control procedures', for the baseline, post-educational and post-promotional campaign samples, in the two hospitals

Hospital	Baseline	Post-education campaign	Post-promotion campaign
Experimental	49.84 (181)	50.26 (114)	50.45 * (148)
Control	50.30 (158)	49.89 (152)	50.41 * (135)

* Changes not statistically significant

Table 9.3 Mean scores on factor one, 'appraisal of, and willingness to comply with, infection control procedures', for the baseline, post-educational and post-promotional campaign samples, by occupational group, in the two hospitals

Occupational group	Baseline	Post-education campaign	Post-promotion campaign
Experimental hospital			
Surgeons	50.42 (24)	49.46 (13)	51.33 (18)
Physicians	50.48 (21)	51.11 (18)	50.90 (30)
Other medical specialists	50.13 (13)	50.36 (11)	49.69 (16)
Nurses	49.50 (105)	50.18 (72)	50.24 (84)

(continued)

Occupational group	Baseline	Post-education campaign	Post-promotion campaign
Control hospital			
Surgeons	45.40 (5)	47.10 (10)	47.78 (9)
Physicians	47.60 (15)	47.45 (11)	50.06 (16)
Other medical specialists	50.06 (18)	49.37 (41)	51.32 (25)
Nurses	50.88 (120)	50.74 (90)	50.48 (85)

The only significant source of variation was between the occupational groups in the two hospitals. However there was no significant difference between scores on factor one between the two hospitals after the promotional campaign, between occupational groups in the two hospitals after the promotional, nor after the educational campaign.

Mean scores were computed for factor two: *appraisal (cost / benefit) of infection control* for the two hospitals' baseline, post-educational and post-promotional campaign data, and also between occupational groups. An analysis of variance was computed to test the significance of any difference between the means. These data are presented in Tables 9.4 and 9.5.

Table 9.4   Mean scores on factor two, 'appraisal of infection control procedures', for the baseline, post-educational and post-promotional campaign samples, in the two hospitals

Hospital	Baseline	Post-education campaign	Post-promotion campaign
Experimental	9.63 (181)	8.94 (114)	9.94 * (148)
Control	8.89 (158)	9.13 (152)	9.30 * (135)

* Changes not statistically significant

Table 9.5   Mean scores on factor one, 'appraisal of infection control procedures', for the baseline, post-educational and post-promotional campaign samples, by occupational group, in the two hospitals

Occupational group	Baseline	Post-education campaign	Post-promotion campaign
Experimental hospital			
Surgeons	10.00 (24)	10.54 (13)	11.28 (18)
Physicians	11.05 (21)	10.33 (18)	10.33 (30)
Other medical specialists	9.06 (13)	8.64 (11)	10.63 (16)
Nurses	9.43 (105)	8.35 (72)	9.38 (84)

(continued)

Occupational group	Baseline	Post-education campaign	Post-promotion campaign
Control hospital			
Surgeons	9.60 (5)	10.40 (10)	10.08 (9)
Physicians	8.80 (15)	8.55 (11)	9.06 (16)
Other medical specialists	9.94 (18)	9.05 (41)	9.92 (25)
Nurses	8.72 (120)	9.09 (90)	9.09 (85)

The only significant source of variation was between the occupational groups. There was no significant difference between scores on factor two after the promotional campaign, or between occupational groups after the promotional or educational campaign, in the two hospitals.

(b) *Conclusion*

From the above results it can be seen that neither the educational nor the promotional campaign were effective in changing the attitudes of staff, primarily the nursing staff, in the Experimental hospital.

9.3 Knowledge questionnaire

The knowledge questionnaire was re-administered to medical and nursing staff in both hospitals following the educational and promotional campaigns in the Experimental hospital. The number of medical and nursing staff completing the questionnaire at each stage are shown in Table 9.1. Again it can be seen that while the majority of nurses completed the questionnaire at each stage, only a small proportion of the doctors did do.

(a) *Results*

i) Analysis of total scores. The mean total scores for the two hospitals and by occupational group were calculated (Tables 9.6 and 9.7). An analysis of variance was also performed to test the significance of differences between the means.

Table 9.6 Mean total scores on the knowledge questionnaire, for the baseline, post-educational and post-promotional campaign samples, in the two hospitals

Hospital	Baseline	Post-education campaign	Post-promotion campaign
Experimental	62.96 (183)	65.42 * (111)	67.02 * (151)
Control	65.11 (151)	64.55 (145)	63.60 (135)

* Statistically significant increase, when compared with baseline

There was a significant difference between the two hospitals and between the occupational groups. There was also a significant difference between occupational groups in the two hospitals. Most importantly, there was a significant difference between the two hospitals over time: staff in the Experimental hospital showed an increased total knowledge score after both the educational campaign and promotional campaign, in comparison with the baseline value. This increase was mainly due to improvements in the nurses' scores in the Experimental hospital.

Table 9.7 Mean total scores on the knowledge questionnaire for the baseline, post-educational and post-promotional campaign samples, by occupational group, in the two hospitals

Occupational group	Baseline	Post-education campaign	Post-promotion campaign
Experimental hospital			
Surgeons	70.33 (24)	70.46 (13)	70.48 (18)
Physicians	69.92 (26)	71.82 (17)	71.94 (30)
Other medical specialists	70.18 (28)	72.77 (13)	72.98 (17)
Nurses	57.63 (105)	61.46 (68)	63.41 (86)
Control hospital			
Surgeons	71.80 (5)	68.10 (10)	70.78 (8)
Physicians	70.53 (17)	70.25 (8)	69.76 (13)
Other medical specialists	69.69 (16)	68.83 (41)	69.41 (23)
Nurses	63.35 (113)	61.57 (86)	61.29 (90)

ii) Analysis of the knowledge questionnaire *sections mean scores.* The mean scores on each of the five knowledge sections were compared for the baseline, post-educational and post-promotional campaigns in the two hospitals. Analysis of variance was used to test the significance of differences between means. These data are presented in Table 9.8.

Table 9.8 *Mean scores on the five sections of the knowledge questionnaire, for the baseline, post-educational and post-promotional campaign samples*

Questionnaire	Hospital	Baseline	Post-education campaign	Post-promotion campaign
Section 1 *Properties of* *microorganisms*	Experimental Control	6.27 7.01	6.61 * 7.28	6.66 * 6.96
Section 2 *Transmission of* *microorganisms*	Experimental Control	8.66 9.07	8.70 9.01	8.76 9.10
Section 3 *Aseptic and hygienic* *techniques*	Experimental Control	9.58 10.05	10.10 * 9.62	10.29 9.65
Section 4 *General knowledge* *of cross-infection*	Experimental Control	13.22 13.52	14.19 * 13.54	14.53 * 13.62
Section 5 *Infectious diseases*	Experimental Control	11.44 11.13	11.25 11.08	11.39 11.37

* Statistically significant difference, when compared with baseline

There was a significant difference between the means on section (1), *properties of micro-organisms*, for occupational groups between the two hospitals. In addition, there was a significant difference between the two hospitals, particularly over time: staff in the Liverpool hospital gained a higher score on this section after the educational campaign and this was maintained after the promotional campaign; staff in the London hospital did not. There were no significant differences between the occupational groups after the promotional campaign.

The significant sources of variation on section (2), *transmission of micro-organisms*, were between hospitals, occupational groups and occupational groups in the two hospitals. However, there were no significant differences in the knowledge scores on this section either by occupational groups, or hospitals, after the interventions.

The significant sources of variation on section (3), *aseptic and hygienic techniques*, were between occupational groups and occupational groups in the two hospitals. There was also a significant difference between the two hospitals over time: staff in the Experimental hospital scored higher on section three after both the educational and promotional campaigns compared with base-line; staff in the Control hospital did not.

The significant sources of variation on section (4), *general knowledge of cross-infection*, were between the occupational groups and occupational groups in the two hospitals. There was also a significant difference between the two hospitals over time: staff in the Experimental hospital scored higher on this section after the educational campaign and again after the promotional campaign compared with baseline; staff in the Control hospital did not.

The only significant source of variation on section (5), *knowledge of infectious diseases*, was between the occupational groups. There were no differences due to the interventions.

(b) *Conclusion*

Unlike attitudes, knowledge of hospital-acquired infections and their control was significantly affected by the educational and promotional campaigns in the Experimental hospital.

9.4 Handwashing frequency

Handwashing frequency was measured in a gynaecological clinic and an orthopaedic ward at the Experimental hospital, following the educational campaign; and in the orthopaedic ward, following the implementation of various phases of the promotional campaign. These data are presented in Table 9.9

Table 9.9 Handwashing frequency during the baseline, post-educational and post-promotional campaigns, in the experimental hospital

Phase	Orthopaedic ward		Gynaecological clinic	
	Number of days	Handwashes per nurse per shift	Number of days	Handwashes per nurse per shift
1 Baseline	21	5.54	21	7.34
2 Post-education campaign	22	4.80	18	9.22
3 Post-promotion campaign				
❑ *Introduction of new soap*	14	6.72	N / A	N / A
❑ *Distribution of video film and educational leaflets*	15	8.10	N / A	N / A
❑ *Television and radio publicity*	14	8.21	N / A	N / A
4 Follow-up after six-months	14	5.57	N / A	N / A

N / A = not assessed

110

From Table 9.9 the following patterns can be ascertained:

- the handwashing frequency showed no increase as a consequence of the educational campaign, but

- increases in handwashing frequency occurred following the promotional campaign;

- these gains were lost by the time of the follow-up, six months later.

9.5 Summary

Neither the educational nor the promotional campaign was effective in changing the attitudes of staff in the Control hospital. This may be due to the fact that staff attitudes were generally fairly positive and appropriate prior to the intervention campaigns (i.e. a 'ceiling' effect); or simply to the nature of the interventions.

The educational (informational) campaign led to a significant increase in total score on the knowledge questionnaire in the Experimental hospital. This increase was maintained following the promotional campaign.

The knowledge questionnaire changes in the Experimental hospital were prominent in three out of the five sections, namely: *properties of micro-organisms, aseptic and hygienic techniques* and *general knowledge of cross-infection.*

Handwashing behaviour, in terms of frequency changes, was not affected by the educational (informational) campaign. The handwashing frequency however, as measured in one of the trial areas, did show a significant increase (i.e. virtually doubled) following the three components of the promotional campaign.

The improvements in handwashing frequency following the promotional campaign had disappeared six months later.

Chapter Ten

THE CONTRIBUTION OF PSYCHOLOGY TO THE CONTROL OF HOSPITAL INFECTIONS: SUMMARY AND CONCLUDING THOUGHTS

10.1 The perennial problem

The history of the prevention of hospital-acquired infections (HAI) illustrates many changes in direction, brought about as different problems arose, and how some measures introduced to curtail the spread of HAI created unexpected new risks. In the mid-1800s it was the application of antiseptics and the introduction of aseptic techniques, that reduced post-operative mortality rates substantially. Antibiotics in the 1930-40s successfully controlled the spread of streptococcal infections, predominant at that time. Further antibiotic expansion heightened the optimism that the problem of infection was about to be resolved for ever. However, antibiotic-resistant organisms, often more virulent than their antibiotic-susceptible progenitors, started emerging gradually. Epidemics and endemics of HAI, caused by previously unheard of organisms, increasingly refractory to treatment, became common. In the 1980's multiply-resistant organisms such as *Staphylococcus aureus* typified the new kind of common infections that cannot be treated with antibiotics. Numerous patients are succumbing to such infections, in spite of the plethora of antibiotics available. Moreover, the progress made in sophisticated therapeutic regimens and the increasingly invasive diagnostic techniques, particularly in surgery (e.g. organ transplantation, joint replacements, etc.), are impaired by increased risks of unmerited infection. At the same time, the potency of improved immunosuppressive drugs has created a new underclass of patients, the 'compromised', who are exceedingly susceptible to infections.

One in ten patients in English hospitals acquires an infection whilst in hospital. These commonly affect the lower respiratory and urinary tract; post-operatively soft tissues may become septic. Patients with HAI stay in hospital longer; an average of 13 days (Freeman, Rosner & McGowen, 1979); they also tend to receive more antibiotics and additional supportive medication. Estimates of the cost of HAI have been given in Chapter One.

10.2 Traditional approaches to the control of hospital-acquired infections

Infection control measures, such as thorough aseptic techniques, judicious use of antibiotics, effective skin antisepsis, regular ward disinfection, organised supply of disposable / sterile materials and carefully programmed infection surveillance have all had some success in controlling HAI. The USA SENIC Report (Chapter One) showed that surveillance was effective in lowering infection rates but any success must be judged in terms of rates balanced against risks (Haley et al., 1980). Whilst rates of HAI have not improved in recent decades, the overall capability to counteract such infections with new antibiotics has not interrupted medical progress. Antibiotics have also allowed considerable advances in organ transplantation. However, in the development of infection control programmes, personal factors have been largely overlooked. For example, one study showed that of 61 programmes, only one centred on social control measures (Wahba, 1977). The full potential of some measures may not have been realised because of a human failure to apply them to their maximum effect. Thus psychology has, potentially, a great deal to contribute to the effective control of this perennial problem. The psychological approach concentrates on people rather than the environment and focuses specifically on staff awareness, a pertinent understanding of fundamental knowledge and adherence to established preventative practices. Few psychological investigations have been conducted this area: status differences (Bromley, 1983; Raven & Haley, 1982), role models (Laufman, 1983; Larson, 1983a) and factors influencing handwashing behaviour (Larson & Killien, 1982) have been the only contributions to date.

10.3 An assessment of the knowledge and attitudes of clinical staff

The present study was aimed at assessing the knowledge and attitudes of hospital staff towards infection control and their adherence to relevant measures. After extensive pilot work and revision of the research instruments (Chapters Four and Five), the underlying attitudes and knowledge of doctors and nurses in an Experimental and a Control university hospital were examined, establishing a baseline against which the effects of subsequent interventions in the Experimental hospital could be evaluated. Mean differences in scores of the attitude questionnaire showed that certain questions were answered significantly differently in the two hospitals. Questions endorsed more highly in the Control hospital reflected differences between medical and nursing staff: for example, nurses were more likely to agree that *more training in infection control is needed for medical staff.* Differences in emphasis, concerning responsibility for cross-infection, produced higher endorsement of the statement that *the ward sister should be held principally responsible for any cross-infection which occurs on her ward,* in the Control hospital. Only one question was given greater endorsement in the Experimental hospital, namely *constant handwashing, use of aseptic techniques, etc. is bad for the hands.* This may reflect differences in washing facilities, soap, etc. between the two hospitals.

Analysis of two factors, (1) *Appraisal and willingness to comply* and (2) *Appraisal of infection control,* extracted during analysis of the pilot study data, showed no significant baseline differences between the two hospitals on either (Chapter Four). There were, however, some occupational group differences: surgeons in the Experimental hospital had a significantly more positive attitude towards factor one than in the Control hospital; and nurses in the latter were significantly more positive towards this factor than their counterparts in the Experimental hospital. Physicians in the Experimental hospital were significantly more positive in their attitudes to factor two than their colleagues in the Control hospital.

Analysis of mean scores on each of four *a priori* categories showed that nurses from the Control hospital scored significantly higher on the education category (more of whom had received special infection control education), and on the perception category, than did nurses in the Experimental hospital. Furthermore, physicians in the latter hospital scored significantly higher their colleagues in the Control hospital on the appraisal category. Examination of differences in knowledge scores in the two hospitals produced a pattern of differences on specific knowledge items, which made sense when the relative training emphasis and the likely differences in experience of infections at these hospitals were taken into account. Overall there were no significant differences between the two hospitals' total mean knowledge scores. All categories of medical staff had similar scores to each other. Nurses had a significantly lower mean knowledge score than doctors. In general, nurses at the Experimental hospital scored significantly lower than their counterparts in the Control hospital.

Analysis of scores on the five knowledge sections demonstrated that nurses in the Control hospital scored significantly higher than those in the Experimental hospital on most of the sections; except on the infectious diseases section, in which there was no difference. There were no significant differences between the medical groups on any of the sections, except the infectious diseases section, where medical specialists in the Control hospital scored significantly higher than those in the Experimental hospital. This particular section required specialist knowledge of communicable diseases, as shown by the lower scores of other doctors not familiar with these diseases (Chapter Five).

10.4 Why are hands still not being washed ?

Handwashing was singled out as the hallmark of standard infection control procedures and studied in detail. Although handwashing is considered the most important single procedure for preventing HAI, at least two reports have exposed poor compliance with handwashing protocols, especially by physicians in intensive care units (Albert & Condie, 1981) and by staff nursing patients under containment isolation (Larson, 1983b). Lapses in handwashing present a complex problem that may be caused by lack of motivation, or lack of knowledge, about the importance of handwashing. It may also be caused by factors such as understaffing, inconveniently located washbasins, absence of paper towels, a harsh-to-the-skin soap, or dermatitis experienced previously by handwashing. A longitudinal handwashing study was carried out to identify which of these factors, alone or in combination, contribute significantly to the problem of low compliance with standard recommendations.

The baseline handwashing frequency (5-8 per shift) in the two clinical areas studied was very much lower than that which would be expected if staff were handwashing 20-30 times per shift, as recommended by most authorities (CDC, 1985). The handwashing frequency, monitored according to the location of washbasins, showed the majority of handwashes to be performed in relatively 'public' areas. This suggests that social factors (e.g. peer pressure) and convenience may play an important role in determining when and where staff do handwash.

Not surprisingly, self-reports of personal handwashing frequency did not match with the actual (observed) frequency. Staff tended to overestimate, by approximately three times, their actual frequency. This discrepancy suggests that most are aware that they should handwash frequently. Their practices, however, indicate that they fail to apply correct knowledge.

The educational campaign failed to produce any increase in handwashing frequency, although knowledge was improved in the Experimental hospital. This supports the contention that correct knowledge is not always followed by the appropriate application of infection control procedures. There was, in fact, a slight decrease in handwashing frequency after the educational campaign. A confounding variable, 'time of year', is a likely cause for that reduction in handwashing frequency: cold weather can cause skin dryness and may discourage staff from handwashing frequently. The frequency was monitored after each of a three-component promotional campaign interventions. It was noted that, even though measurements were collected during the winter months, a significant improvement in handwashing frequency was achieved following the promotional campaign. The introduction of a specially formulated soap and handwashing promotion posters (first intervention) produced an increase; the release of a handwashing training video and educational leaflets (second intervention) produced a further and more substantial improvement; after the publicity campaign (third intervention) the handwashing frequency did not rise again but remained at the higher level achieved by the second intervention.

From the above findings it is possible to conclude that poor compliance with handwashing protocols is caused neither by lack of knowledge about the importance of handwashing *per se*, nor by obstacles such as inconveniently located wash basins. Poor compliance is caused by a lack of motivation, although the seasonal variation suggests a 'skin condition' deterrent. If staff are motivated, as occurred during the promotional campaign, their handwashing frequency increases. However a six month follow-up study indicated that motivation was short-lived. The improved behavioural compliance had returned to its baseline level.

Handwashing technique, measured by the area washed when using a 'disclosing' dye instead of water, was poor among nursing staff. Sixty-five percent of nurses missed some part of the hand surface, commonly the finger tips: the area which is most likely to come into contact with patients or the inanimate environment. The techniques of nurses after the educational campaign were not significantly different from baseline: 60% still missed some part of the hand surface. However, after the promotional handwashing campaign, only 35% missed some part of the hand surface.

When tested for hand carriage of micro-organisms, a majority of staff showed high numbers of normal microflora, suggesting infrequent handwashing. Many carried strict pathogens such as *Staphylococcus aureus*. When asked to predict what organisms might be present on their hands, during 'clean' activities, well over half did actually expect some pathogenic organisms to be present; half, indeed, did carry potential pathogens on their hands. However, in only 9 of 28 subjects who anticipated carriage of organisms, did their prediction prove to be correct. Many, though expecting pathogens to be present, carried on regardless with their clinical work, without handwashing. The probable presence of organisms did not seem to influence behaviour.

The handwashing frequency of senior doctors during ward rounds was disappointing: only two instances of handwashing were observed during 21 hours of observation. Neither the educational nor the promotional campaign succeeded in improving medical compliance with standard practices. This was probably due to the reluctance of doctors to spend time watching the handwashing training video or reading the educational materials (or to perform handwashing !). These findings emphasise the necessity for increasing the compliance of all doctors with such elementary practice, perhaps by incorporating such procedures into the medical undergraduate curriculum (Chapter Six).

10.5 Is it the soap ?

In order to rectify one possible reason for low compliance, namely the deterrent effect of a low quality handwashing product, a special soap was formulated to the preferred specifications of the Experimental hospital staff. Trials with this 'optimal soap' showed that handwashing frequency was higher than with other prototype formulations (natural or synthetic), and only fractionally lower than the mean baseline frequency on a trial ward. On a trial clinic, the handwashing frequency with the optimal soap was greater than with a soap of natural formulation but less than with a synthetic soap and even less than the baseline frequency. These variations in frequency may have been due to seasonal affecting factors. However, it appears that overall handwashing frequency was not greatly influenced by the availability of a quality, mild hand-cleanser, especially formulated according to the preferences of staff themselves (Chapter Seven).

An assessment of 11 selected nursing priorities showed that nurses deemed *patient comfort* as their most important priority, the *administration of medicines* as their second and *infection control* as a last priority (E.E. Williams, unpublished data). Thus, in theory, infection control was perceived as an important aspect of nursing duties. This, however, conflicted with the opinion expressed in the attitude questionnaire that the main reason for non-compliance with infection control procedures was *lack of time*. If *infection control* was indeed a high priority, its application should not be abandoned when staff are busy.

A questionnaire which required nurses to rank handwashing priorities (E.E. Williams, unpublished data) showed they had a logical understanding of basic infection control knowledge and, although there were some anomalies, the order in both hospitals was similar to the priorities ranked by infection control experts. This again illustrates the point that lack of knowledge is not a major reason for low compliance with infection control procedures.

The study of nursing activities in the intensive care unit indicated a considerable range (2-20) in the frequency of handwashing per shift of 6.5 hours; the average frequency of 8.4 was much lower than expected. Staff rarely practised alcohol hand-rubbing and, in general, appeared confused about its correct use. Large numbers of micro-organisms were present on staffs' hands during routine patient duties and no clear distinction could be made between tasks which transferred 'more' or 'less' organisms.

The standard guidelines for handwashing were compared with actual staff practices to ascertain to what extent they adhered to these guidelines before and after a special educational seminar. Before the seminar, handwashing was observed before and after dressing surgical wounds in only 40% of cases; and after touching inanimate sources likely to be contaminated in 39% of cases. Handwashing for these two indications was greatly improved after the educational seminar. Before the seminar, situations involving, for example, handling of body fluids, excretions, etc., and where infection risks were obvious (e.g. invasive procedures) were accompanied by the highest handwashing compliance; that is, when an indication was readily recognised as important. Overall, before the seminar, there was compliance in over half (57.1%) of the situations where handwashing was indicated. After the seminar, handwashing for all indications was improved, with the exception of handwashing after exposure to body fluids, where handwashing was increased to 75.4% of all necessary handwashes. In addition, the increased use of alcoholic hand disinfectants was gratifying. Thus, following intensive instruction by a senior member of the infection control staff, a significant improvement was produced. The feasibility, however, of conducting such seminars throughout the hospital, as a matter of routine, is questionable.

Although *busyness* was given as the major reason for lack of compliance with infection control procedures, no inverse relationship was noted between handwashing frequency and number of activities: that is, handwashing did not decrease during busy periods. In fact, as the activity level increased, so did the handwashing frequency. There was no evidence to support the claim that lack of handwashing was due to lack of time. (Chapter Eight).

10.6 Is it lack of education ?

The educational campaign was designed to impart theoretical knowledge of infections and their control, and specific information concerning practical applications. The three main posters on disinfection, antisepsis and isolation were seen by 30% of doctors and 50% of nurses interviewed; those who had referred to them had obtained the information they required. All staff who were asked about *isolation precautions* had consulted the posters and found them useful. This indicates that staff prefer simple and direct instructions rather than more theoretical and detailed information. Such instructions may also have acted as reminders of the isolation recommendations.

Analysis of the two factors of the attitude questionnaire showed no differences in either factor, in the two hospitals, before and after the educational campaign. The four *a priori* categories studied also showed no significant differences before and after the educational campaign in the two hospitals. Thus the educational campaign, aimed mainly at influencing staff knowledge of infection control, failed to improve staff attitudes.

The reasons given by staff in the Control hospital, as being responsible for cross-infection, were the same before and after the educational campaign. However, in the Experimental hospital both *the patient* and *food* were given more 'blame' after the campaign. The principal reason stated, however, *hands and clothes of hospital staff* did not change. The demotion of *fomites* (i.e. contaminated articles) to a lower order of importance may be explained by a perception amongst staff that, because detailed information on disinfection had become widely available, fomites were less likely sources of infection.

The reasons given for failing to comply with hygienic measures remained the same in both hospitals before and after the educational campaign. *Shortage of time* was still the most popular reason, followed by *confusion* and *forgetting*.

In order to establish a standard against which to measure the knowledge scores of hospital staff, a preliminary sample of non-hospital staff was studied, their overall mean score was 57.80 out of a possible 84. Analysis of the total knowledge scores of hospital staff showed a significant difference between the two hospitals before and after the educational campaign. The Experimental hospital sample produced a significant increase in total score in comparison with the Control hospital. Furthermore, each of the four occupational groups in the Experimental hospital exhibited a higher mean total knowledge score after the campaign than before. The highest increase was achieved by the nurses, who scored 3.83 points above their baseline score .

Staff in the Experimental hospital scored significantly higher after the educational campaign on sections (1) *properties of micro-organisms*, (3) a*septic and hygienic techniques* and (4) *general knowledge of cross-infection.* Occupational differences were noted between scores on *aseptic and hygienic techniques*; physicians and nurses from the Experimental hospital scored higher after the campaign than before. Section (3) is particularly relevant to nursing staff, as the majority of their daily activities necessitates a high standard of aseptic and hygienic techniques. It is therefore especially significant that nurses in the Experimental hospital showed improved knowledge in this area (Chapter Nine).

In conclusion, the educational campaign did improve theoretical knowledge of HAI. Although it has been shown that educational campaigns can improve knowledge, this *per se* does not necessarily lead to the application of such knowledge. As shown by the behavioural measures previously discussed, there was no 'post-educational campaign' increase in compliance with established infection control practices.

There could be several explanations for the lack of compliance with isolation procedures, handwashing, and other fundamental infection control practices. Staff may feel that they are not personally susceptible to HAI, that such infections are not serious, or that control measures are not effective deterrents to their spread. A health belief questionnaire (Becker *et al.*, 1977), with a section concerning each of these three areas, was designed. It was completed by 113 of 600 clinical staff who were invited to respond. Since, however, many respondents had personally experienced a HAI (48.7%), that sample was biased (E.E. Williams, unpublished data). Personal experience was, in fact, noted to have a significant influence on the subjects' attitude to HAI. Those with personal experience of HAI perceived themselves as more susceptible, the infections as more serious and preventive measures as more effective, than staff with no such experience. The latter finding is somewhat surprising: it may be the case that those who did not apply preventive measures to their patients and who have not been previously exposed to HAI, may regard such precautions as unnecessary. It does appear that one reason for non-compliance is that staff do not think they are susceptible to HAI and, therefore, do not think it necessary to take preventive measures. The frequency distributions on this question were greatly skewed towards the *not susceptible* end of the scale. Nurses were significantly more likely to perceive themselves as susceptible than were doctors. They were also significantly more likely to perceive infections as serious. Naturally, nurses have greater contact with patients and are therefore more likely to witness the consequences of HAI. If an infection is seen as serious, control procedures are believed to be useful in its prevention. It is possible to predict that, as doctors perceive themselves less susceptible to personal infection and also perceive such infections to be less serious, they would be less likely to comply with control measures. Staff with personal experience of a HAI would also be more likely to implement infection control measures in future, than would those without such an experience.

10.7 Is it lack of awareness ?

The promotional campaign was designed to motivate and encourage staff to comply with infection control procedures. An optimal soap (to minimise one possible deterrent to handwashing), handwashing promotional posters, a handwashing training video tape, educational leaflets and publicity were all key components in the campaign. Again there were no significant differences in the attitude scores, between the two hospitals, on the two factors concerning *appraisal* and *willingness to comply*, before and after the promotional campaign. The four *a priori* categories, education, compliance, perception of infection risks and appraisal also failed to show any differences in the two hospitals, before and after the campaign .

The reasons given as responsible for cross-infection also remained unaffected by the promotional campaign. Reasons stated by staff in the Experimental hospital, for failing to comply with hygienic measures, changed slightly: *shortage of time* was still given as the major reason for non-compliance. However, *forgetting* fell from second to fourth place after the promotional campaign. Hence the campaign may, at least, have acted as a reminder for the application of aseptic and hygienic techniques.

Overall, an extensive promotional campaign produced no significant attitudinal change in the Experimental hospital. As discussed in previous chapters, attitudes are influenced by many factors and have a complex relationship with knowledge and behaviour. The behavioural change seen after the promotional campaign, since it was not accompanied by a corresponding attitude change, may have been superficial and thus was short-lived.

The effect of the promotional campaign on knowledge was, however, significant: staff in the Experimental hospital improved their mean total knowledge score after the educational campaign and again after the promotional campaign. Scores on the three knowledge sections, which had shown significant improvement in the Experimental hospital following the educational campaign *(properties of micro-organisms, aseptic and hygienic techniques* and *general knowledge of cross-infection)*, remained significantly improved after the promotional campaign.

10.8 There is a lack of issue-relevant thinking

The psychological approach to the control of HAI is concerned with ways of enhancing the awareness of infection control amongst staff, focusing on the influence of personal factors and motivating individuals to adopt high standards of practice.

The educational and promotional campaigns did result in an increased knowledge of infection control. The latter also brought about a significant behavioural change, in terms of improved compliance with handwashing recommendations. Both campaigns, however, failed to ensure a long-term change in attitude. Their failure to evoke a lasting change may account for the temporary nature of the improvement in behavioural compliance. This suggests that future studies should address the issue of how best to bring about permanent changes in attitude, in addition to improvements in knowledge and behaviour.

One other possible interpretation of our results can be formulated in terms of the Elaboration Likelihood Model (ELM; Petty & Cacciopo, 1986). In Chapter Eight, when describing the rationale behind the promotional campaign, we indicated that we deliberately sought to use a broad based approach in order to appeal to staff at various levels. According to the ELM, a strategic approach to the control of HAI should involve both the central and peripheral routes to persuasion (Bartzokas & Slade, 1991). Thus we aspired to encourage staff to think about the problem and importance of handwashing, as well as emotionally appealing to them to handwash. The educational video tape on handwashing, probably the most successful component in the campaign, was designed to inform and to encourage 'issue-relevant thinking', thus operating *via* the central route to persuasion. The promotional posters on handwashing were specifically designed to make an 'emotional appeal', thus operating *via* a peripheral route. The fact that behaviour change was not permanent, indicates that the effect of the campaigns was more peripheral than central. That is, they worked well at the level of emotional appeal, stimulating temporary improvements in handwashing, but failed to engage centrally sufficient numbers of staff in 'issue-relevant thinking' over a sufficiently long period of time, to bring about a permanent behavioural change.

10.9 Concluding thoughts

Awareness of the importance of preventing infection must be ingrained in the undergraduate curriculum of all health care staff. The principal aim of any educational campaign should be to supplement and reinforce a deeply entrenched knowledge, not to substitute for basic teaching. If outbreaks of hospital sepsis necessitate the belated education of staff in elementary principles of infection control, veiled as an 'educational campaign', it is a sad reflection on the values and priorities of undergraduate teaching.

Infection pervades every single hospital activity. It is only through diligent hygienic practices that the sick can be protected from hazards of infection and allowed time to heal. In the judicious implementation of hygiene nothing counts more than thinking. Microorganisms, however, being 'out of sight' also remain 'out of mind'. The fragrance of disinfectants in an apparently 'clean' hospital environment seems to attenuate mental vigilance and to divert attention away from focusing on the vectors of microbial transmission towards partaking in a variety of rituals of dubious value. As a result, staff become confused over priorities. The importance of personal responsibility, highlighted in this study, has not been recognised, to date.

The guidelines that formed the basis of our educational campaign were specially designed by professional typographers for accessibility, clarity of presentation and maximum psychological impact. Despite such diligent preparations, the resulting behavioural improvements were short-lived. What is the value of medical education and postgraduate training if these cannot elicit the correct behaviour in practice ?

We do not claim that a psychological approach by itself can resolve the perennial problem of HAI. We have here merely outlined early attempts to probe the psyche of doctors and nurses, in the belief that the key to preventing HAI lies therein. Clinical psychologists, when describing patients who do not follow doctors' orders, refer to 'non-compliance'. What term can one use for doctors, who by disregarding the fundamental tenets of hygiene, harm their patients? Is negligence too strong an epithet for such aberrant behaviour?

Health care staff are, by and large, self-motivating, from 'within'. Incentives are possibly one way to achieve a permanent improvement in the practice of hospital hygiene. But should such a tactic be deemed necessary for professional people? How can professionals be encouraged to do their duty from 'without'? The time has come to expose those who heal with one hand and, literally harm with the other.

REFERENCES

Abraham, E.P. (1980). 'Fleming's Discovery'. *Review of Infectious Diseases* **2**, p. 140.

Ackerknecht, E. H. (1982). *A Short History of Medicine*, John Hopkins University Press, Baltimore.

Ajzen, I. & Fishbein, M. (1980). *Understanding Attitudes and Predicting Social Behaviour*, Englewood-Cliffs, NJ. Prentice-Hall.

Albert, R. K. & Condie, F. (1981). 'Handwashing Patterns in Medical Intensive Care Units.' *New England Journal of Medicine* **304**, pp. 1465-1466.

Alkateeb, W., Lukeroth, C. J. & Riggs, M. (1975). 'A Comparison of Three Educational Techniques Used in a Venereal Disease Clinic.' *Public Health Reports* **90**, pp. 159-164.

Altemeier, W. A. (1979). 'Surgical Infections: Incisional Wounds.' In: *Hospital Infections* (Bennett, J.V. & Brachman, P.S., Eds.), Little Brown, Boston.

American Hospital Association (1974). 'Committee on Infections within Hospitals, Statement on Microbiologic Sampling in the Hospital.' *Journal of the American Hospital Association* **48**, pp. 125-156.

Ayliffe, G. A. J., Babb, J. R., Bridges, K., *et al.* (1975). 'Comparison of Two Methods for Assessing the Removal of Total Organisms and Pathogens from the Skin.' *Journal of Hygiene (Cambridge)* **75**, pp. 259-274.

Ayliffe, G. A. J., Collins, B. J. & Taylor, L. J. (1982). *Hospital-acquired Infection, Principles and Prevention*, John Wright & Sons, Bristol.

Ayliffe, G. A. J. & Taylor, L, J. (1984). 'Preface in Proceedings of the First International Conference of Infection Control.' *Journal of Hospital Infection* **5** (Suppl. A), pp. vii-viii.

Ayliffe, G.A.J., Lowbury, E.J.L., Geddes, A.M. & Williams, J.D. (Eds.) (1992). *Control of Hospital Infection: A practical handbook.* Chapman & Hall Medical, London.

Bailey, J. L. (1974). 'Contraceptive Pamphlets in Colombian Drugstores.' *Studies in Family Planning* 5, pp. 178-182.

Barber, M. (1947). 'Staphylococcal Infection Due to Penicillin-resistant Strains.' *British Medical Journal* ii, p. 863.

Bartzokas, C. A., Paton, J. H., Gibson, M. F., Graham, R., McLoughlin, G. A. & Croton, R. S. (1984). 'Control and Eradication of Methicillin-resistant *Staphylococcus aureus* on a Surgical Unit.' *New England Journal of Medicine* 311, pp. 1422-1425.

Bartzokas, C.A., Gibson, M.F., Graham, R. & Pinder, D.C. (1983). 'A Comparison of Triclosan and Chlorhexidine Preparations with 60% Isopropyl alcohol for Hygienic Hand Disinfection.' *Journal of Hospital Infection* '4, pp. 245-255.

Bartzokas, C.A. & Slade, P.D. (1991). 'Motivation to comply with infection control procedures.' *Journal of Hospital Infection* 18 (Suppl. A), pp. 508-514.

Becker, M. H., Maiman, L. A., Kirscht, J. P., Haefner, D. P. & Drachman, R. H. (1977). 'The Health Belief Model and Prediction of Dietary Compliance: a Field Experiment.' *Journal of Health and Social Behaviour* 18 (4), pp. 348-366.

Beland, I. L. & Passos, J. Y. (1975). 'Problems with Infections.' In: *Clinical Nursing, Pathophysiological and Psychosocial Approaches* (3rd ed.), Macmillan, New York.

Benenson, A.S. (Ed.) (1975). *Control of Communicable Diseases in Man* (12th Ed.), American Public Health Association, Washington.

Berman, R. & Knight, R. (1969). 'Evaluation of Hand Antisepsis.' *Archives of Environmental Health* 18, pp. 781-783.

Blackwell, C. C. & Weir, D. M. (1981). *Principles of Infection and Immunity in Patient Care,* Churchill Livingstone, London.

Bradley, J. M., Noone, P., Townsend, D. E. & Grubb, W. B. (1985). 'Methicillin-resistant *Staphylococcus aureus* in a London Hospital.' *Lancet* **351**, pp. 1493-1495.

Bromley, D. (1983). 'Psychological Factors in Hospital Infection.' *Journal of Infection Control Nursing* **23** (Suppl.), pp. 11-14.

Broughall, J. M., Marshman, C., Jackson, B. & Bird, P. (1984). 'An Automatic Monitoring System for Measuring Handwashing Frequency in Hospital Wards.' *Journal of Hospital Infection* **5**, pp. 447-453.

Brown, J. P. (1969). 'A Study of Posters in Dental Health Education.' *Australian Dental Journal* **14**, pp. 312-318.

Bryan, C. S. & Deever, E. (1981). 'Implementing Control Measures.' *American Journal of Infection Control* **9** (4), pp. 101-105.

Casewell, M. W. & Phillips, I. (1977). 'Hands as Routes of Transmission for *Klebsiella* species.' *British Medical Journal* **2**, pp. 1315-1317.

Centers for Disease Control (1983). *Guidelines for Prevention and Control of Nosocomial Infections,* US Department of Health and Human Services, Hospital Infections Program, Atlanta.

Centers for Disease Control (1985). *Guideline for Handwashing and Hospital Environmental Control.* (Revised by J.S. Garner & M.S. Favero), US Department of Health and Human Services, Hospital Infections Program, Atlanta.

Chaiken, S. & Stangor, C. (1987). 'Attitudes and Attitude Change.' *Annual Review of Psychology* **38**, pp. 575-630.

Chain, E., Florey, H.W., Gardner, A.D. *et al.* (1940). 'Penicillin as a Chemotherapeutic Agent.' *Lancet* **2**, p. 226.

128

Child, D. (1976). *The Essentials of Factor Analysis,* Rinehart & Winston, London.

Clarke, W. D., Devine, M., Jolly, B. C. & Meyrick, R. L. (1977). 'Health Education with a Display Machine in the Surgery.' *Health Education Journal* 36 (4), pp. 100-113.

Collee, J. G. (1976). *Applied Medical Microbiology,* Blackwell, Oxford.

Cooper, J. & Croyle, R.T. (1984). 'Attitudes and Attitude Change.' *Annual Review of Psychology* 35, pp. 395-426.

Cruickshank, R., Duguid, J. P., Marmion, B. P. & Swain, R. H. A. (1973). *Medical Microbiology. A Guide to the Laboratory Diagnosis and Control of Infection,* Churchill Livingstone, London.

Cruse, P. J. E. & Foord, R. (1973). 'A Five-year Prospective Study of 23,649 Surgical Wounds.' *Archives of Surgery* 107, pp. 206-210.

Dixon, R. E. (1978). 'Effect of Infections on Hospital Care.' *Annals of Internal Medicine* 89 (2), pp. 749-753.

Dowling, H. F. (1959). 'The History of the Broad Spectrum Antibiotics.' *Antibiotic Annual* 39, pp. 1958-1959.

Dubay, E. C. & Grubb, R. D. (1978). *Infection, Prevention and Control* (2nd ed.), C. V. Mosby & Co., St. Louis.

Eickhoff, T. C. (1977). 'Perspectives in Hospital Infection.' In: *Infection Control in Health Care Facilities* (Cundy, K.R. & Ball, W., Eds.), University Park Press, Baltimore.

Emerton, M. D. (1976). *Principles and Practice of Nursing,* University of Queensland Press, Queensland.

Evans, C. A., Smith, W. M., Johnston, E. A. & Giblett, E. R. (1950). 'Bacterial Flora of the Normal Human Skin.' *Journal of Investigative Dermatology* 15, pp. 305-314.

Evans, C. A. & Stevens, R. J. (1976). 'Differential Quantitation of Surface and Subsurface Bacteria of Normal Skin by the Combined Use of the Cotton Swab and the Scrub Method.' *Journal of Clinical Microbiology* **3** (6), pp. 576-581.

Fahlberg, W. J. & Groschel, D. (1978). *Occurrence, Diagnosis and Sources of Hospital-Associated Infections,* Marcel Dekker Inc., Basel.

Farquhar, J. W., Wood, P. D., Breitrose, H., *et al.* (1977). 'Community Education for Cardiovascular Health.' *Lancet* **i**, pp. 1192-1195.

Fazio, R.H. (1986). 'How do attitudes guide behaviour?'. In *The Handbook of Motivation and Cognition: Foundations of Social Behaviour* (Sorrentino R.M. & Higgins E.T., Eds.), NY, Guilford Press.

Feldman, H. (1969). 'Learning Transfer from Programmed Instruction to Clinical Performance.' *Nursing Research* **18** (1), pp. 51-54.

Finland, M. (1970). 'Changing Ecology of Bacterial Infections as Related to Antibacterial Therapy.' *Journal of Infectious Diseases* **122**, pp. 419-431.

Fleming, A. (1929). 'On the Antibacterial Action of Cultures of a Penicillium with Special Reference to their use in the Isolation of *B. influenzae.*' *British Journal of Experimental Pathology* **10**, p. 226

Freeman, J., Rosner, B. A. & McGowen, J. E. (1979). 'Adverse Effects of Nosocomial Infection.' *Journal of Infectious Diseases* **140** (5), pp. 732-740.

Gatherer, A., Parfit, J., Poser, E. & Vessey, M. (1979). *Is Health Education Effective?* The Health Education Council, London.

Goldman, M. (1987). *Lister Ward.* Adam Hilger, London.

Goodier, T. E. W. & Parry, W. R. (1959). 'Sensitivity of Clinically Important Bacteria to Six Common Antibacterial Substances.' *Lancet* **i**, p. 356.

Gordon, A. M. (1980). 'Gentamicin-resistant Klebsiella Strains in Hospital.' *British Medical Journal* **1**, pp. 722-723.

Gould, D. (1985). 'Don't Spread that Infection...Theoretical Knowledge of Infectious Diseases' *Nursing Mirror*, **161** (4), pp. 52-53.

Gould, J. C. (1958). 'Environmental Penicillin and Penicillin-Resistant *Staphylococcus aureus*.' *Lancet* **i**, p. 489.

Griffiths, L. R., Bartzokas, C. A., Hampson, J. P. & Ghose, A. R. (1986). 'Antibiotic Prescribing Patterns in a Recently Commissioned Liverpool Teaching Hospital. Part 1 Treatment.' *Journal of Hospital Infection* **8** (2), pp. 159-167.

Haefner, D. P. & Kirscht, J. P. (1970). 'Motivational and Behavioural Effects of Modifying Health Beliefs.' *Public Health Report* **85**, pp. 478-484.

Haley, R. W., Quade, D., Freeman, H. E. *et al.* (1980). 'Study on the Efficacy of Nosocomial Infection Control (SENIC Project). Summary of Study Design.' *American Journal of Epidemiology* **111**, pp. 472-485.

Haley, R. W. & Shachtman, R. H. (1980). 'The Emergence of Infection Surveillance and Control Programmes in US Hospitals: an Assessment.' *American Journal of Epidemiology* **111**, pp. 574-591.

Haley, R. W., Hightower, A. W., Khabbaz, R. F., *et al.* (1982). 'The Emergence of Methicillin-Resistant *Staphylococcus aureus* Infections in US Hospitals.' *Annals of Internal Medicine* **97**, pp. 297-308.

Hann, J. B. (1973). 'The Source of the Resident Flora'. *The Hand* **5** (3), pp. 247-252.

Hart, C. A. (1982). 'Nosocomial Gentamicin and Multiply-resistant Enterobacteria at One Hospital. 1 Description of an Outbreak.' *Journal of Hospital Infection* **3**, pp. 15-28.

Hewitt, W. L. & Sanford, J. P. (1974). 'Workshop on Hospital-associated Infections.' *Journal of Infectious Diseases* **130** (6), pp. 680-686.

Hill, D. J. (1978). 'Simple Health Education about Breast Cancer in General Practice.' *International Journal of Health Education* **21**, pp. 124-126.

Himmelsbach, C. K. (1966). 'The physician's Role in Hospital Infection Control.' *General Practice* **33**, pp. 103-107.

Hinton, N. A. (1971). 'Why Infection Control Programs Fail.' *Canadian Hospital* **77**, pp. 48-49 & 77.

Holmes, O. W. (1936). 'On the Contagiousness of Puerperal Fever. Puerperal Fever as a Private Pestilence.' *Medical Classics* **1** (3), Williams & Wilkins, Baltimore.

Hooton, T. M., Haley, R. W., Culver, D. H., White, J. W. & Morgan, W. M. (1981). 'The Joint Associations of Multiple Risk Factors with the Occurrence of Nosocomial Infection.' *American Journal of Medicine* **70**, pp. 960-970.

Jackson, G. C. (1974). 'Perspective from a Quarter Century of Antibiotic Usage.' *Journal of the American Medical Association* **227**, pp. 634-637.

Kipnis, D., Schmidt, S. & Wilkinson, I. (1980). 'Intraorganizational Influence Tactics: Explorations in Getting One's Way.' *Journal of Applied Psychology* **65**, pp. 440-452.

Kirscht, J. P. (1973). 'Effects of Repeated Threatening Health Communications.' *International Journal of Health Education* **16**, p. 268.

Kornhauser, A. & Sheatsley, P. B. (1976). 'Questionnaire Construction and Interview Procedure.' In: *Research Methods in Social Relations* (Selltiz, C., Wrightsman, L.S. & Cook, S.W., Eds.) Holt, Rinehart & Winston, New York.

Larson, E. (1981). 'Persistent Carriage of Gram-negative Bacteria on Hands.' *American Journal of Infection Control* **9**, pp. 112-119.

Larson, E. & Killien, M. (1982). 'Factors Influencing Handwashing Behaviour of Patient Care Personnel.' *American Journal of Infection Control* **10**, pp. 93-99.

Larson, E. (1983a). 'Influence of a Role Model on Handwashing Behaviour.' *American Journal of Infection Control* **11** (4), p. 146.

132

Larson, E. (1983b). 'Compliance with Isolation Technique.' *American Journal of Infection Control* **11** (6), pp. 221-225.

Larson, E. (1984). 'Current Handwashing Issues.' *Infection Control* **5** (1), pp. 15-17.

Larson, E., McGinley, K. J., Grove, G. L., Leyden, J. J. & Talbot, G. V. (1986). 'Physiologic, Microbiologic, and Seasonal Effects of Handwashing on the Skin of Health Care Personnel.' *American Journal of Infection Control* **14** (2), pp. 51-59.

Laufman, H. (1983). 'Infection Control: a Moral Issue.' *Today's OR Nurse* **5** (7), pp. 38-46.

Legler, D. W., Gilmore, R. W. & Stuart, G. C. (1971). 'Dental Education of Disadvantaged Adult Patients: Effects of Dental Knowledge and Oral Health.' *Journal of Periodontics* **42** (9), pp. 565-570.

Leventhal, H., Singer, R. & Jones, S. (1965). 'Effects of Fear and Specificity of Recommendation Upon Attitudes and Behaviour.' *Journal of Personality and Social Psychology* **2** (1), pp. 20-29.

Lowbury, E. J. L., Lilly, H. A. & Bull, J. P. (1964). 'Disinfection of Hands: Removal of Transient Organisms.' *British Medical Journal* **2**, pp. 230-233.

Major, R. H. (1954). *A History of Medicine 2*, Charles C. Thomas, Illinois.

Maki, D. G. (1978). 'Control of Colonisation and Transmission of Pathogenic Bacteria in the Hospital.' *Annals of Internal Medicine* **89**, 5(2), pp. 777-780.

McDonald, P. J. (1982). 'Methicillin-resistant Staphylococci: a Sign of the Times ?' *Medical Journal of Australia* **1**, pp. 445-446.

McGowan, J. E. & Finland, M. (1974). 'Infection and Antibiotic Usage at Boston City Hospital: Changes in Prevalence During the Decade 1964-1973.' *Journal of Infectious Diseases* **129**, pp. 421-428.

133

McGowen, J. E. (1982). 'Cost and Benefit - a Critical Issue for Hospital Infection Control.' *American Journal of Infection Control* **10** (3), pp. 100-108.

McLane, C., Chenelly, S., Sylwestrak, M. L. & Kirchhoff, K. T. (1983). 'A Nursing Practice Problem : Failure to Observe Aseptic Technique.' *American Journal of Infection Control* **11** (5), pp. 178-182.

Mildner, R., Ohgke, H. & Pfefferhorn, T. M. (1984). *System of Hand Hygiene, Scientific Principles and Optimal Use in Practice.* Rohrberg & Mildner, Hamburg.

Moncrieff, R. W. (1966). *Odour Preference.* Leonard Hill, London.

Moore, M. M. & Abbott, N. K. (1980). 'Accountability Translated into Action: Handwashing.' *National Intravenous Therapy Association* **3** (1), pp. 13-22.

Mortimer, E. A., Wolinsky, E., Gonzaga, A. J. & Rammelkamp, C. H. (1966). 'Role of Airborne Transmission in Staphylococcal Infections.' *British Medical Journal* **1**, pp. 319-322.

Neu, H. C. (1978). 'How is the Medical Student Being Trained in Microbiology and Infections?' *Annals of Internal Medicine* **89** (2), pp. 818-820.

Noble, W. C. & Lidwell, O. M. (1963). 'Environmental Contamination.' In: *Infection in Hospitals, Epidemiology and Control.* (Williams, R.E.O. & Shooter, R.A., Eds.), Blackwell, Oxford.

Ojajarvi, J., Makela, P.& Rantasalo, I. (1977). 'Failure of Hand Disinfection with Frequent Handwashing: a Need for Prolonged Field Studies.' *Journal of Hygiene* (Cambridge) **79**, pp. 107-112.

Ojajarvi, J. (1981). 'The Importance of Soap Selection for Routine Hand Hygiene in Hospital.' *Journal of Hygiene* (Cambridge) **86**, pp. 275-283.

Olson, I. A. (1970). 'Advantages and Disadvantages of Closed-Circuit Television in the Teaching of Large Classes in Preclinical Medicine.' *British Journal of Medical Education* **4**, pp. 312-315.

Oppenheim, A. N. (1979). *Questionnaire Design and Attitude Measurement.* Basic Books, New York.

Palmer, M. B. (1984). *Infection Control, a Policy and Procedure Manual.* W. B. Saunders & Co., Philadelphia.

Paterson, R. & Aitken-Swan, J. (1958). 'Public Opinion on Cancer, Changes Following Five Years of Cancer Education.' *Lancet* **2**, pp. 791-793.

Perlitsh, M. J. (1974). 'Seven Warnings of Gum Disease: an Evaluation of a Pamphlet Designed to Educate the Public.' *Journal of Periodontology* **45**, p. 542.

Petty, R.E. & Cacioppo, J.T. (1986). 'The Elaboration Likelihood Model of Persuasion.' *Advances in Experimental Social Psychology* **19**, pp. 123-205.

Pratkanis, A.R. & Greenwald, A.G. (1989). 'A Socio-cognitive Model of Attitude Structure and Function.' *Advances in Experimental Social Psychology* **22**, pp. 245-285.

Price, P. B. (1938). 'The Bacteriology of Normal Skin.' *Journal of Infectious Diseases* **63**, pp. 301-318.

Raven, B. H., Freeman, H. E. & Haley, R. W. (1982). 'Social Science Perspectives in Hospital Infection Control.' In: *Contemporary Health Services Social Science Perspectives* (Johnson, A. W., Grusky, O. & Raven, R.H., Eds.), Auburn House, Massachusetts.

Raven, B. H. & Haley, R. W. (1982). 'Social Influence and Compliance of Hospital Nurses with Infection Control Policies.' In: *Psychology and Behavioural Medicine.* (Eiser, J.R., Ed.), J.S. Wiley & Sons, London.

Rines, A. R. & Montag, M. L. (1976). *Nursing Concepts and Nursing Care.* J.S. Wiley & Sons, New York.

Rosen, M. J. (1970). *An Evaluative Study Comparing the Cognitive and Attitudinal Effect of Two Versions of an Educational Programme About Mind-affecting Drugs (Final report)*. Evaluation & Research Associates, Los Angeles.

Sawyer, W. D., Kapral, F. A., Knight, V., Manire, G. P. & Paterson P. Y. (1978). 'Microbiology and Immunology Curricula for Medical Students.' *American Society of Microbiology News* 44, pp. 190-195.

Scanlon, J. W. & Leikkanen, M. (1973). 'The use of Fluorescein Powder for Evaluating Contamination in a Newborn Nursery.' *Journal of Pediatrics* 82, pp. 966-971.

Seto, W.H., Ching, T.Y., Ng, S.H., Chu, Y.B. & Ong, S.G. (1988). 'The application of Influencing Tactics in Infection Control: a Study on Staff Compliance.' *Proceedings of the Second International Conference on Infection Control*, Harrogate.

Shooter, R. A. (1965). 'The Environment.' In: *Skin Bacteria and Their Role in Infection.* (Maibach, H.I. & Hildick-Smith, G., Eds.), McGraw-Hill, New York.

Singer, C. & Underwood, E. A. (1962). *A Short History of Medicine.* Clarendon Press, Oxford.

Spitznagel, A. (1969). 'Behaviour Change through Health Education: Problems of Methodology.' *Proceeding of the First International Seminar*, World Health Organisation, Federal Centre for Health Education, Hamburg.

Sprunt, K., Redman, W. & Leidy, G. (1973). 'Antibacterial Effectiveness of Routine Handwashing.' *Pediatrics* 52, pp. 264-271.

Taylor, L. J. (1978). 'An Evaluation of Handwashing Techniques (Part 1).' *Nursing Times* 74, pp. 54-55.

Tesser, A. & Shaffer, D.R. (1990). 'Attitudes and Attitude Change.' *Annual Review of Psychology* 41, pp. 479-523.

Thompson, R. L. & Wenzel, R. P. (1982). 'International Recognition of Methicillin-resistant Strains of *Staphylococcus aureus.*' *Annals of Internal Medicine* **97**, pp. 925-926.

Updegraff, D. M. (1964). 'A Culture Method of Quantitatively Studying the Microorganisms of the Skin.' *Journal of Investigative Dermatology* **42** (2), pp. 129-137.

Wahba, A. H. W. (1977). 'Hospital Infections: a Continuing Danger to Patients and Staff.' *World Health Organisation Chronicle* **31**, pp. 63-66.

Walker, R. M. (1963). 'Definition of the Problem.' In: *Infection in Hospitals, Epidemiology and Control.* (Williams, R.E.O. & Shooter, R.A., Eds.), Blackwell, Oxford.

Wenzel, B. M. (1948). 'Techniques in Olfactometry: a Critical Review of the Last 100 Years.' *Psychological Bulletin* **45**, pp. 231-247.

Wenzel, R.P. (Ed.) (1993). *Prevention and Control of Nosocomial Infections.* (2nd Edition), Williams & Wilkins, Baltimore.

Williams, J. D. (1984). 'Antibiotic guidelines.' *British Medical Journal* **288**, pp. 343-344.

Winner, H. I. (1978). *Microbiology in Patient Care.* Hodder & Stoughton, London.

Winnick, C. (1963). 'Tendency systems and the effects of a movie dealing with a social problem'. *Journal of General Psychology* **68**, 289 - 305.

Wolff, L., Weitzel, M. H. & Fuerst, E. V. (1979). *Fundamentals of Nursing.* J. P. Lippincott & Co., Philadelphia.

Zimakoff, J., Stormark, M. & Larsen, S.O. (1988a). 'Multicentre Investigations of Hand Hygiene Behaviour Among Staff in Intensive Care Units in Two Hospitals in Denmark and Two Hospitals in Norway.' *Proceedings of the Second International Conference on Infection Control*, Harrogate.

Zimakoff, J., Kjelsberg, A.B., Larsen, S.O. & Holstein, B. (1988b). 'A Multicentre Investigation of Attitudes to Hand Hygiene Assessed by Staff in Twelve Hospitals in Denmark and Three in Norway.' *Proceedings of the Second International Conference on Infection Control*, Harrogate.

ATTITUDES TO CROSS INFECTION SCALE

QUESTIONNAIRE

Age [   ]   **Occupation** Surgeon
                                     Physician
Sex [   ]   Microbiologist
                                     Other medical specialist
                                     Nurse
                                     Domestic
                                     Other clinical staff

✓
[   ]
[   ]
[   ]
[   ]
[   ]
[   ]
[   ]

Please indicate the extent to which you *agree* or *disagree* with each of the following statements by circling one of the numbers below it.

1   Now that antibiotics are more readily available, preventive measures are less important.

Strongly disagree	Disagree	Uncertain	Agree	Strongly agree
-2	-1	0	+1	+2

2   Some infection control procedures are too demanding to strictly adhere to.

Strongly disagree	Disagree	Uncertain	Agree	Strongly agree
-2	-1	0	+1	+2

3   More training in infection control is needed for nursing staff.

Strongly disagree	Disagree	Uncertain	Agree	Strongly agree
-2	-1	0	+1	+2

4   More training in infection control is needed for medical staff.

Strongly disagree	Disagree	Uncertain	Agree	Strongly agree
-2	-1	0	+1	+2

5   The instruction I have been given on infection control has been useful.

Strongly disagree	Disagree	Uncertain	Agree	Strongly agree
-2	-1	0	+1	+2

6   Hospital infection courses are only necessary for infection control nurses and microbiologists, not all hospital staff.

Strongly disagree	Disagree	Uncertain	Agree	Strongly agree
-2	-1	0	+1	+2

7   The ward sister should be held principally responsible for any cross-infection which occurs on her ward.

Strongly disagree	Disagree	Uncertain	Agree	Strongly agree
-2	-1	0	+1	+2

8   Patients are right to expect high hygiene standards even if the staff must spend more time on each procedure.

Strongly disagree	Disagree	Uncertain	Agree	Strongly agree
-2	-1	0	+1	+2

9   If a doctor / nurse suspects a colleague of an unhygienic practice he / she should explain the error to them.

Strongly disagree	Disagree	Uncertain	Agree	Strongly agree
-2	-1	0	+1	+2

10   It is necessary for doctors / nurses to read current literature on infection control relevant to their work.

Strongly disagree	Disagree	Uncertain	Agree	Strongly agree
-2	-1	0	+1	+2

11   All doctors / nurses should attend occasional refresher courses in infection control to maintain standards.

Strongly disagree	Disagree	Uncertain	Agree	Strongly agree
-2	-1	0	+1	+2

12   Continued assessment and implementation of necessary changes would be useful in control of infection.

Strongly disagree	Disagree	Uncertain	Agree	Strongly agree
-2	-1	0	+1	+2

13   Even if all hospital staff observed the correct procedures wherever necessary, cross-infection would not be significantly reduced.

Strongly disagree	Disagree	Uncertain	Agree	Strongly agree
-2	-1	0	+1	+2

14   Little can be done to further reduce cross-infection.

Strongly disagree	Disagree	Uncertain	Agree	Strongly agree
-2	-1	0	+1	+2

15 Hospital patients are very susceptible to cross-infection.

Strongly disagree	Disagree	Uncertain	Agree	Strongly agree
-2	-1	0	+1	+2

16 Hospital-acquired infections cause only minor illnesses.

Strongly disagree	Disagree	Uncertain	Agree	Strongly agree
-2	-1	0	+1	+2

17 It is not feasible to maintain good hygiene procedures in a large hospital.

Strongly disagree	Disagree	Uncertain	Agree	Strongly agree
-2	-1	0	+1	+2

18 The current infection control procedures in this hospital are effective.

Strongly disagree	Disagree	Uncertain	Agree	Strongly agree
-2	-1	0	+1	+2

19 Strict adherence to control of infection procedures is a luxury which the busy nurse / doctor can seldom afford.

Strongly disagree	Disagree	Uncertain	Agree	Strongly agree
-2	-1	0	+1	+2

20 Constant handwashing, use of aseptic techniques, etc. is bad for the hands.

Strongly disagree	Disagree	Uncertain	Agree	Strongly agree
-2	-1	0	+1	+2

Please tick any of the following which you feel are responsible for hospital cross-infection.

✓

1	The patient	☐
2	Hands and clothes of hospital staff	☐
3	Instruments / dressings	☐
4	Food	☐
5	Fomites (bedpans / blankets, etc.)	☐

Please tick any of the following which you feel are responsible for the non-use of hygienic methods.

6	Shortage of time	☐
7	Poor washing facilities (soap / wash basins)	☐
8	Confusion over correct procedure	☐
9	Not necessary	☐
10	Forgetting	☐

Have you had any formal training in infection control? ☐

Appendix Two

CROSS INFECTION KNOWLEDGE

QUESTIONNAIRE

	✓
Age ☐	**Occupation** Surgeon ☐
	Physician ☐
Sex ☐	Microbiologist ☐
	Other medical specialist ☐
	Nurse ☐
	Domestic ☐
	Other clinical staff ☐

Please answer the following questions by circling either *true, false* or *don't know*.

1   'Hospital bacteria' have the same
    sensitivity to antibiotics as
    'community bacteria'.   *True*   *False*   *Don't know*

2   Viruses are the group of
    microorganisms most likely to cause
    a severe hospital-acquired infection.   *True*   *False*   *Don't know*

3   Chemical disinfection is the best way
    of sterilising surgical instruments.   *True*   *False*   *Don't know*

4   Most bacteria are capable of
    producing disease in man.   *True*   *False*   *Don't know*

5   Viruses can only grow in living cells.   *True*   *False*   *Don't know*

6   Fungi cause infection mainly in
    immunosuppressed patients.   *True*   *False*   *Don't know*

7	Once a specimen, e.g. urine, is collected from a patient it can be stored on the ward for several days before microbiological tests.	*True*	*False*	*Don't know*
8	Bacteria can only enter the body through the respiratory tract or breaks in the skin.	*True*	*False*	*Don't know*
9	If a person does not show signs or symptoms of disease he / she cannot pass on the disease.	*True*	*False*	*Don't know*
10	Infectious diseases can be spread only by direct contact.	*True*	*False*	*Don't know*
11	Injections can transmit infections.	*True*	*False*	*Don't know*
12	If a nurse's hands are visibly clean he / she cannot spread infection.	*True*	*False*	*Don't know*
13	Shedding skin scales is a way of spreading microbes.	*True*	*False*	*Don't know*
14	Gastrointestinal infections are mainly spread by faeces or contaminated food.	*True*	*False*	*Don't know*
15	The single most important measure in the prevention of hospital cross-infection is efficient handwashing.	*True*	*False*	*Don't know*
16	All patients with an infection need to be isolated.	*True*	*False*	*Don't know*
17	Avoiding frequent wound exposure helps to reduce cross-infection.	*True*	*False*	*Don't know*
18	Alcohol is an efficient disinfectant when rubbed into the skin.	*True*	*False*	*Don't know*
19	The non-touch technique is used only to change dressings or infected wounds.	*True*	*False*	*Don't know*
20	Protective isolation is necessary for patients with most forms of immunodeficiency.	*True*	*False*	*Don't know*

21	Antiseptic solutions applied to the hands kill organisms immediately.	True	False	Don't know
22	The aim of handwashing, on wards, is to remove the transient organisms.	True	False	Don't know
23	About 5-10% of all patients get an infection once they are in hospital.	True	False	Don't know
24	Although antibiotics may effectively control an infection, they can also make the patient vulnerable to other infections.	True	False	Don't know
25	A notifiable infection is one which is usually fatal.	True	False	Don't know
26	In the early stages of bacterial infection there is often a higher white cell count than normal.	True	False	Don't know
27	All people are susceptible to infection to the same extent.	True	False	Don't know
28	Wearing a mask prevents transmission of airborne microbes.	True	False	Don't know
29	The incidence of hospital-acquired infections has decreased since the introduction of antimicrobial drugs.	True	False	Don't know
30	Urinary tract infections are one of the most common forms of hospital-acquired infections.	True	False	Don't know
31	Colonisation is when organisms grow on a person without producing a reaction.	True	False	Don't know
32	The presence of pus is a reliable sign of wound infection.	True	False	Don't know
33	Pulmonary tuberculosis is a rare notifiable infection in Great Britain today.	True	False	Don't know
34	The commonest site of infection in typhoid fever carriers is the gall bladder.	True	False	Don't know

35   Urinary tract infections are usually caused by Gram-negative bacilli.

True   False   Don't know

36   Measles requires one week's isolation from the onset of the rash.

True   False   Don't know

37   Only cows can get anthrax.

True   False   Don't know

38   Herpes zoster can lead to chicken pox in non-immune contacts.

True   False   Don't know

39   Whooping cough only becomes infectious from the onset of coughing.

True   False   Don't know

40   Staphylococci easily become resistant to fucidin or rifampicin.

True   False   Don't know

41   Rubella has its most serious effects in non-immune males.

True   False   Don't know

42   Poliomyelitis is not infectious.

True   False   Don't know

STUDIES IN HEALTH AND HUMAN SERVICES